Management of Intraoperative Crises

Editor

SHANDA H. BLACKMON

THORACIC SURGERY CLINICS

www.thoracic.theclinics.com

Consulting Editor
M. BLAIR MARSHALL

August 2015 • Volume 25 • Number 3

ELSEVIER

1600 John F. Kennedy Boulevard • Suite 1800 • Philadelphia, Pennsylvania, 19103-2899

http://www.thoracic.theclinics.com

THORACIC SURGERY CLINICS Volume 25, Number 3
August 2015 ISSN 1547-4127, ISBN-13: 978-0-323-39358-4

Editor: John Vassallo (j.vassallo@elsevier.com)
Developmental Editor: Susan Showalter

Thoracic Surgery Clinics (ISSN 1547-4127) is published quarterly by Elsevier Inc., 360 Park Avenue South, New York, NY 10010-1710. Months of publication are February, May, August, and November. Business and editorial offices: 1600 John F. Kennedy Boulevard, Suite 1800, Philadelphia, PA 19103-2899. Periodicals postage paid at New York, NY, and additional mailing offices. Subscription prices are $350.00 per year (US individuals), $453.00 per year (US institutions), $165.00 per year (US Students), $435.00 per year (Canadian individuals), $585.00 per year (Canadian institutions), $225.00 per year (Canadian and international students), $465.00 per year (international individuals), and $585.00 per year (international institutions). Foreign air speed delivery is included in all Clinics' subscription prices. All prices are subject to change without notice. **POSTMASTER:** Send address changes to Thoracic Surgery Clinics, Elsevier Health Sciences Division, Subscription Customer Service, 3251 Riverport Lane, Maryland Heights, MO 63043. **Customer Service (orders, claims, online, change of address): Telephone: 1-800-654-2452 (U.S. and Canada); 314-447-8871 (outside U.S. and Canada). Fax: 314-447-8029. E-mail: journalscustomerservice-usa@elsevier.com (for print support); journalsonlinesupport-usa@elsevier.com (for online support).**

Reprints. For copies of 100 or more, of articles in this publication, please contact Commercial Rights Department, Elsevier Inc., 360 Park Avenue South, New York, NY 10010-1710. Tel: 212-633-3874; Fax: 212-633-3820; E-mail: reprints@elsevier.com.

Thoracic Surgery Clinics is covered in *MEDLINE/PubMed (Index Medicus), EMBASE/Excerpta Medica, Science Citation Index Expanded (SciSearch®), Journal Citation Reports/Science Edition,* and *Current Contents®/Clinical Medicine*.

Contributors

CONSULTING EDITOR

M. BLAIR MARSHALL, MD, FACS
Chief, Division of Thoracic Surgery; Associate Professor of Surgery, Department of Surgery, Georgetown University Medical Center, Georgetown University School of Medicine, Washington, DC

EDITOR

SHANDA H. BLACKMON, MD, MPH, FACS
Associate Professor, Division of Thoracic Surgery, Department of Surgery, Mayo Clinic, Rochester, Minnesota

AUTHORS

MARK F. BERRY, MD
Associate Professor, Department of Cardiothoracic Surgery, Falk Cardiovascular Research Center, Stanford University, Stanford, California

BRYAN M. BURT, MD, FACS
Assistant Professor, Division of General Thoracic Surgery, Michael E. DeBakey Department of Surgery, Baylor College of Medicine, Houston, Texas

JORDY C. COX, MD
UCSF Department of Cardiothoracic Surgery, UCSF Medical Center, San Francisco, California

MARCELO CYPEL, MD
Assistant Professor, Division of Thoracic Surgery, Toronto General Hospital, University Health Network, University of Toronto, Toronto, Ontario, Canada

SETH FORCE, MD
Chief, General Thoracic Surgery; The Andrew J. McKelvey Professor of Lung Transplantation; Associate Professor of Surgery, Division of Cardiothoracic Surgery, Emory University Hospital, Emory University School of Medicine, Atlanta, Georgia

ERIC L. GROGAN, MD, MPH, FACS
Assistant Professor, Department of Thoracic Surgery, Tennessee Valley Healthcare System, Nashville Campus, Vanderbilt University Medical Center, Nashville, Tennessee

SHAWN S. GROTH, MD, MS
Assistant Professor, Division of General Thoracic Surgery, Michael E. DeBakey Department of Surgery, Baylor College of Medicine, Houston, Texas

DAVID M. JABLONS, MD
Professor and Chief Thoracic Surgery, UCSF Department of Surgery, Nan T. McEvoy Distinguished Professor of Thoracic Surgical Oncology, Ada Distinguished Professor of Thoracic Oncology, Program Leader Thoracic Oncology, UCSF Helen Diller Comprehensive Cancer Center, San Francisco, California

SHAF KESHAVJEE, MD
Professor, Division of Thoracic Surgery, Toronto General Hospital, University Health Network, University of Toronto, Toronto, Ontario, Canada

NATALIE LUI, MD
Clinical Fellow, Division of Thoracic Surgery, Harvard Medical School, Massachusetts General Hospital, Boston, Massachusetts

TIAGO N. MACHUCA, MD
Fellow, Division of Thoracic Surgery, Toronto General Hospital, University Health Network, University of Toronto, Toronto, Ontario, Canada

ROBERT J. McKENNA Jr, MD
Division of Thoracic Surgery, Department of Surgery, Cedars-Sinai Medical Center, Los Angeles, California

HEATHER MERRY, MD
Division of Thoracic Surgery, Department of Surgery, Cedars-Sinai Medical Center, Los Angeles, California

KATIE S. NASON, MD, MPH
Division of Thoracic and Foregut Surgery, Department of Cardiothoracic Surgery, University of Pittsburgh, Pittsburgh, Pennsylvania

MANU SANCHETI, MD
Assistant Professor of Surgery, Division of Cardiothoracic Surgery, Emory St. Joseph's Hospital, Emory University School of Medicine, Atlanta, Georgia

INDERPAL S. SARKARIA, MD, FACS
Department of Cardiothoracic Surgery, University of Pittsburgh Medical Center, Pittsburgh, Pennsylvania

DEREK SERNA-GALLEGOS, MD
Division of Thoracic Surgery, Department of Surgery, Cedars-Sinai Medical Center, Los Angeles, California

K. ROBERT SHEN, MD
Associate Professor of Surgery, Division of General Thoracic Surgery, Mayo Clinic, Rochester, Minnesota

DAVID J. SUGARBAKER, MD
Professor and Chief, Division of General Thoracic Surgery, Michael E. DeBakey Department of Surgery, Baylor College of Medicine, Houston, Texas

MATHEW THOMAS, MD
Assistant Professor of Surgery, Division of Cardiothoracic Surgery, Mayo Clinic, Jacksonville, Florida

MANUEL VILLA, MD
Department of Cardiothoracic Surgery, University of Pittsburgh Medical Center, Pittsburgh, Pennsylvania

CAMERON WRIGHT, MD
Professor of Surgery, Division of Thoracic Surgery, Harvard Medical School, Massachusetts General Hospital, Boston, Massachusetts

SAI YENDAMURI, MD, FACS
Department of Thoracic Surgery, Roswell Park Cancer Institute, Elm and Carlton Streets, Buffalo, New York; Yashoda Hospitals, Hyderabad, Telangana, India

ELENA ZIARNIK, MD
Resident, Department of Thoracic Surgery, Vanderbilt University Medical Center, Nashville, Tennessee

Contents

Preface: Managing Intraoperative Events in Thoracic Surgery ix

Shanda H. Blackmon

Erratum x

Pulmonary Artery Bleeding During Video-Assisted Thoracoscopic Surgery: Intraoperative Bleeding and Control 239

Mark F. Berry

With appropriate planning and operative technique, the risk of pulmonary artery injury and bleeding during video-assisted thoracoscopic surgery (VATS) lobectomy can be minimized. However, the risk cannot be completely eliminated; surgeons should always ensure that they are prepared to manage this situation if it occurs. Although pulmonary artery bleeding can potentially lead to intraoperative disasters, appropriate judgment, management, and control via VATS or conversion to thoracotomy can avoid any impact on either short-term or long-term patient outcomes.

Intraoperative Tracheal Injury 249

Natalie Lui and Cameron Wright

Intraoperative tracheal injury is a rare but potentially devastating complication. Transhiatal esophagectomy should be avoided in patients with proximal esophageal tumors who underwent neoadjuvant therapy, and percutaneous tracheostomy should be avoided in patients with short, thick necks. Early recognition leads to improved outcomes. Patients present with a sudden loss in airway pressure, air leaking into the operative field, or mediastinal and subcutaneous emphysema. Treatment starts with airway control. Primary buttressed repair is recommended, through either a left cervical incision for proximal injuries or a right thoracotomy for distal injuries. Nonoperative management has been used safely in select patients injured during intubation or tracheostomy.

Massive Airway Hemorrhage 255

Sai Yendamuri

Massive hemoptysis is not an uncommon surgical problem. A systematic yet flexible and multidisciplinary approach leads to optimal outcomes. The initial focus should be on stabilizing patients and securing the airway, which should be followed by methods to stop the bleeding, preferably nonsurgical methods. Consideration for definitive therapy should ensue, including surgical therapy for appropriate patients. This review outlines the management of patients with massive hemoptysis from benign and malignant causes.

Great Vessel Injury in Thoracic Surgery 261

Manuel Villa and Inderpal S. Sarkaria

The potential for intraoperative bleeding is inherent to the practice of thoracic surgery due to the presence of multiple vital vascular structures, complex anatomy,

and constant cardiorespiratory motion. Careful and detailed preoperative evaluation and planning, comprehensive review of imaging studies, and a thorough knowledge of the operative procedure, anatomic relationships, and potential complications are of the highest importance in prevention and avoidance of bleeding complications. Preparation with a clear crisis management plan ensures an effective and expedited response when intraoperative bleeding occurs.

Endotracheal Tube Management and Obstructed Airway **279**

Manu Sancheti and Seth Force

Thoracic surgery encompasses a wide array of surgical techniques, most of which require lung isolation for surgical exposure in the pleural cavity; this, in turn, demands an extensive knowledge of respiratory mechanics and modalities of airway control. Likewise, effective treatment of an acute central airway obstruction calls for a systematic approach using clear communication between teams and a comprehensive knowledge of available therapeutic modalities by the surgeon.

Operative and Perioperative Pulmonary Emboli **289**

Jordy C. Cox and David M. Jablons

Intraoperative and perioperative massive pulmonary emboli remain an unusual but well-established cause of death. Improved outcomes rely on a high index of suspicion, prompt recognition, and aggressive intervention. Surgical embolectomy outcomes have improved drastically since its inception as a technique at the turn of the previous century and should be used without hesitation during an intraoperative crisis in which pulmonary embolism has been determined to be the cause. There is an emerging trend toward a more aggressive approach.

Acute Intraoperative Pulmonary Aspiration **301**

Katie S. Nason

Acute intraoperative aspiration is a potentially fatal complication with significant associated morbidity. Patients undergoing thoracic surgery are at increased risk for anesthesia-related aspiration, largely due to the predisposing conditions associated with this complication. Awareness of the risk factors, predisposing conditions, maneuvers to decrease risk, and immediate management options by the thoracic surgeon and the anesthesia team is imperative to reducing risk and optimizing patient outcomes associated with acute intraoperative pulmonary aspiration. Based on the root-cause analyses that many of the aspiration events can be traced back to provider factors, having an experienced anesthesiologist present for high-risk cases is also critical.

Coagulopathy and Anticoagulation During Thoracic Surgery **309**

Mathew Thomas and K. Robert Shen

Coagulopathy and bleeding in thoracic surgery may be compounded by the chronic use of anticoagulants and antiplatelet agents. Timely preoperative cessation and postoperative resumption of these antithrombotic drugs are critical in reducing the risks of perioperative major bleeding and thromboembolism. This article describes the various strategies for the optimal perioperative management of antithrombotics based on individual assessment of each patient and the most recent multisociety guidelines.

Intraoperative thoracic surgical catastrophes may require extracorporeal circulation modes to support the patient while the appropriate repair is made. Teamwork is key and, given the evidence supporting better performance with the use of simulation and surgical-crisis checklists, their use should be encouraged. Anticipation is another important factor because the results of intrathoracic malignancy resection are clearly superior in the setting of planned cardiopulmonary support. In addition, familiarity with the different modes of support that are currently available can direct the decision-making process toward the best option to facilitate resolution of the intraoperative catastrophe with the least related morbidity.

Although mortalities have steadily declined over the last 80 years, morbidity after pneumonectomy remains significant. Appropriate patient selection and a proactive approach to perioperative management are essential to optimizing outcomes after pneumonectomy.

Video-assisted thoracic surgery (VATS) lobectomy has become a standard approach for early stage 1 lung cancer. However, concerns still remain regarding certain clinical situations, such as potential damage to the heart or bypass grafts when VATS is performed after median sternotomy for cardiac surgery. In this article, techniques are described to minimize risk to an internal mammary artery graft during a VATS anatomic pulmonary resection in this group of patients. The article reviews data on VATS after median sternotomy for cardiac surgery and describes techniques to prevent, treat, and mitigate problems in this group of patients. Management of intraoperative crises is also discussed.

Immediate postoperative complications are common after lobectomy. The most effective management of postoperative crises is prevention, which starts with preoperative preparation and patient screening. There are many factors that can be controlled and improved by the patient. Equally important is patient selection, which is influenced by pulmonary function tests, cardiopulmonary reserve, and preexisting comorbidities. After the operation, the care team can also greatly improve outcomes with aggressive cardiopulmonary therapies, ambulation, vigilant monitoring, and frequent assessments of the patient. Prevention strategies can minimize risks; however, when they occur, a proactive approach may minimize the long-term sequelae.

THORACIC SURGERY CLINICS

FORTHCOMING ISSUES

November 2015
Prevention and Management of Postoperative Complications
John D. Mitchell, *Editor*

February 2016
Pulmonary Metastasectomy
Thomas A. D'Amico and
Mark W. Onaitis, *Editors*

May 2016
Innovations in Thoracic Surgery
Kazuhiro Yasufuku, *Editor*

RECENT ISSUES

May 2015
Lung Cancer Screening
Gaetano Rocco, *Editor*

February 2015
Lung Transplantation
Sudish C. Murthy, *Editor*

November 2014
Advanced Lung Cancer: Radical Surgical Therapy
Raja M. Flores, *Editor*

RELATED INTEREST

Surgical Clinics of North America, Volume 95, Issue 2 (April 2015)
Perioperative Management
Paul J. Schenarts, *Editor*
Available at: www.surgical.theclinics.com

Preface

Managing Intraoperative Events in Thoracic Surgery

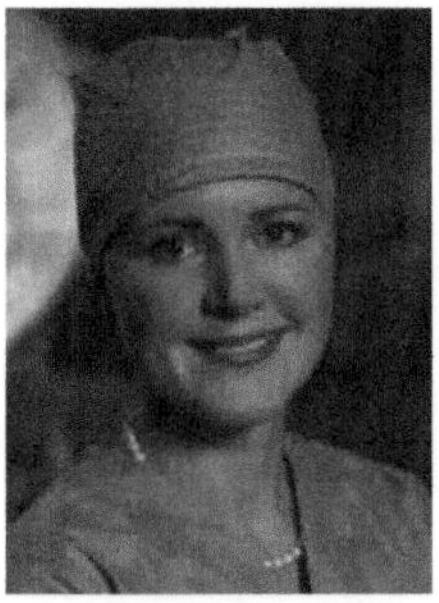

Shanda H. Blackmon, MD, MPH, FACS
Editor

Intraoperative events are best managed when they are avoided or prevented. Unfortunately, some events happen despite the best preoperative preparation. Like airline pilots, surgeons should practice, read about, and rehearse managing intraoperative crises. Team training for these events will result in a better outcome and less morbidity for the patient. As a surgeon, I believe being transparent about outcomes and events leads to better teaching for residents and enhanced learning for everyone involved. Recording every case will allow a surgeon to go back into the event and sometimes identify the critical error and how to best manage or prevent it in the future. Reviewing other surgeons' events can perhaps avoid the event in the future.

Most surgeons remember intraoperative events like they were yesterday, even when they took place years ago. Most of my memories of being a resident in training are punctuated by my mentors constantly reminding me that attention to detail and keeping things simple is the best way to avoid disaster. Dr Garrett Walsh will always be famous for striking fear into the hearts of decades of thoracic surgeons passing through MD Anderson Cancer Center as he would begin to tell the story of a simple intraoperative mistake or event that was not properly managed and then led to another event that eventually sent the patient into a rapid downward spiral death spin. One of my favorite mentors, Dr Bill Putnam, used to always say "fail early." I believe seeing others fail and learning about how they failed and making note of how not to fail in the same manner lead to better outcomes. Our specialty is unique because it is one of the only specialties that still holds open morbidity and mortality conferences. There is nothing more valuable to residents than hearing their surgeon admit to error and state how they may have done things differently.

I hope this issue will live in the operating room instead of the office. Each article was carefully selected based on filling gaps in managing critical events. From complex management of pulmonary artery hemorrhage to intraoperative aspiration, airway crises, and pulmonary embolus, each author has reflected on personal experience as well as reviewed the literature to succinctly deliver management recommendations.

I still remember being in the operating room with Dr Ara Vaporciyan as we encountered a potentially dangerous portion of the surgery. He would lean into the field and remind me how gently one should handle the pulmonary artery or how important it was to place the intercostal muscle over the bronchial stump. After the warning, he would smile and say "Ask me how I know…."

Shanda H. Blackmon, MD, MPH, FACS
Mayo Clinic
200 First Street, Southwest
Rochester, MN 55905, USA

E-mail address:
blackmon.shanda@mayo.edu

Thorac Surg Clin 25 (2015) ix
http://dx.doi.org/10.1016/j.thorsurg.2015.05.001
1547-4127/15/$ – see front matter

Erratum

An error was made in "Esophageal Preservation in Esophageal High-Grade Dysplasia and Intramucosal Adenocarcinoma," in the November 2011 issue of *Thoracic Surgery Clinics*, Volume 21, Number 4, page 527. One of the authors was incorrectly listed as Shah D. Rachit. The author's correct name is Rachit D. Shah.

Thorac Surg Clin 25 (2015) x
http://dx.doi.org/10.1016/j.thorsurg.2015.04.013
1547-4127/15/$ – see front matter

Pulmonary Artery Bleeding During Video-Assisted Thoracoscopic Surgery
Intraoperative Bleeding and Control

Mark F. Berry, MD

KEYWORDS

• Thoracoscopy • VATS lobectomy • Hemorrhage • Complications

KEY POINTS

- Video-assisted thoracoscopic surgery (VATS) lobectomy has been shown to be safe and has many advantages for patients over an approach with a thoracotomy.
- With appropriate planning and operative technique, the risk of pulmonary artery injury and bleeding can be minimized; but surgeons should always ensure that they are prepared to manage this situation if it occurs.
- Pulmonary artery injuries can be repaired via VATS, but surgeons should not hesitate to use conversion to thoracotomy when needed and depending on their VATS experience.

INTRODUCTION

The use of video-assisted thoracic surgery (VATS) dates back to the 1940s when a cystoscope was used to drain a pleural effusion, but it was not until the 1990s when the use of video-assisted techniques to achieve anatomic lung resection such as lobectomy was described.[1] Both single-institution and multi-institution trials have subsequently shown VATS lobectomy to be safe and feasible.[2–4] Controlled studies have also demonstrated benefits of a minimally invasive approach over thoracotomy.[5,6] The technique is particularly beneficial for higher-risk patients, such as older patients and patients with impaired pulmonary function.[7–9] Reports have also documented that a minimally invasive VATS approach can be used in more advanced situations, such as large and central tumors with clinically positive nodal disease and after induction therapy, as well as for sleeve resections, chest wall resections, and pneumonectomy.[10–14]

Despite the advances and demonstrated benefits of minimally invasive thoracic surgery, a VATS approach for lobectomy has not been universally adopted. As recently as 2010, a VATS approach was used in the minority (45%) of lobectomies recorded in the Society of Thoracic Surgeons General Thoracic Surgery Database.[9] Several reasons may explain why a VATS approach has not been more widely used. Despite the advanced applications described earlier, some tumors may still not be technically appropriate for the use of a VATS approach. In addition, some reports have expressed concerns that the lymph node harvest achieved via VATS is inferior to that achieved during thoracotomy.[15–18] However, another significant reason that a VATS approach is not used more often could be concerns that

The author has nothing to disclose.
Department of Cardiothoracic Surgery, Falk Cardiovascular Research Center, Stanford University, 300 Pasteur Drive, Stanford, CA 94305, USA
E-mail address: berry037@stanford.edu

Thorac Surg Clin 25 (2015) 239–247
http://dx.doi.org/10.1016/j.thorsurg.2015.04.007

the ability to safely control and dissect the hilar pulmonary vessels is limited. Some surgeons may not feel comfortable visualizing and handling these structures through a small incision and a scope while watching on a monitor.

In particular, concerns over how to control and repair any inadvertent vascular injury are likely very prominent for many surgeons. Of the pulmonary structures, pulmonary artery bleeding caused by injury during dissection and manipulation is generally the most feared because of the relatively delicate nature of the vessel and very-high-volume blood flow through this structure. Compared with the other hilar pulmonary structures, it is generally thought that the pulmonary artery is most easily injured. Importantly, attempts to repair a pulmonary artery injury can sometimes lead to more extensive tearing that could potentially progress to involve the main pulmonary artery. Major pulmonary artery injuries can result in an intraoperative patient death caused by exsanguination when the injury is not adequately controlled in a timely fashion. Perhaps not as immediately catastrophic but also potentially devastating to patients, a pulmonary artery injury could lead to the need to perform a more extensive pulmonary resection, such as pneumonectomy, rather than the planned lobectomy. The concern over pulmonary artery manipulation during minimally invasive surgery is well captured by an editor's comments about VATS pulmonary resections in a prominent cardiothoracic surgery textbook: "Should a problem occur during a video-assisted procedure when stapling a pulmonary artery branch, I would submit that there will be a significant squeeze on the surgeon's coronary circulation until such time as the chest can be opened."[19]

Reviewing the many successful case series of VATS lobectomy should not lead to an interpretation that potential pulmonary artery bleeding during VATS dissection is insignificant. In contrast, experienced VATS surgeons generally do not understate the importance of safety and careful pulmonary artery manipulation.[20,21] Rather, a more appropriate interpretation of the reported VATS lobectomy series may be that the risk of serious complications resulting from pulmonary artery injuries can be minimized with careful planning and operative technique. The purpose of this article is to review the incidence and mechanisms of pulmonary artery bleeding during VATS lobectomies. In addition, management strategies and techniques to prevent, control, and repair pulmonary artery injuries that occur during VATS procedures is described.

INCIDENCE OF PULMONARY ARTERY BLEEDING DURING VIDEO-ASSISTED THORACOSCOPIC SURGERY LOBECTOMIES

Although concerns over pulmonary artery injuries and bleeding during VATS lobectomy are certainly well founded and understood, estimating the risk and consequences of pulmonary artery injuries during VATS lobectomy is difficult. The incidence of pulmonary artery bleeding reported by large-volume, very experienced surgeons and centers is very low.[4,10,22–27] **Table 1** shows that the incidence of conversion to thoracotomy because of bleeding, which is likely from the pulmonary artery in most cases, ranges from 0.5% to 5.2%. In addition, the reports of an intraoperative catastrophe, such as death, caused by uncontrolled pulmonary artery bleeding in high-volume series are negligible.

However, the incidence of pulmonary artery injuries across the spectrum of surgical experience is likely to be higher than what is reported by higher-volume centers. Instances of pulmonary artery injuries during VATS lobectomy may be underreported in the medical literature, as intraoperative complications are generally not eagerly publicized.

Table 1
Summary of incidence of all conversions and conversions for bleeding in large VATS lobectomy series

	Number of Patients	All Conversions	Conversion for Bleeding
McKenna et al,[4] 2006	1100	28 (2.5%)	6 (0.5%)
Villamizar et al,[10] 2013	916	36 (3.9%)	21 (2.3%)
Puri et al,[23] 2015	604	87 (14.4%)	22 (3.6%)
Liang et al,[25] 2013	382	6 (1.6%)	4 (1.0%)
Roviaro et al,[22] 2004	337	78 (23.1%)	5 (1.5%)
Stephens et al,[24] 2014	307	22 (7.2%)	12 (3.9%)
Samson et al,[26] 2013	193	45 (23.3%)	10 (5.2%)
Nicastri et al,[27] 2008	153	14 (9.2%)	5 (3.3%)

Many surgeons have heard anecdotal tales about significant intraoperative pulmonary artery injuries that were probably never contained in any published series. A vessel injury that is repaired without conversion or any significant patient event may also not be captured or reported. In addition, estimating the occurrence of pulmonary artery bleeding or complications that result from pulmonary artery bleeding during VATS lobectomy in administrative databases can also be difficult, as those cases may be coded as having had a thoracotomy approach if a conversion was performed after the injury. Regardless of the true incidence, all surgeons should maintain the highest level of concern to avoid pulmonary artery bleeding during a VATS lobectomy regardless of their experience.

MECHANISMS OF PULMONARY ARTERY INJURY

During Dissection of an Adjacent Hilar Structure

There are several ways that the pulmonary artery can be inadvertently injured during a VATS lobectomy. One mechanism of injury is during dissection of an adjacent structure, particularly when the pulmonary artery is posterior to a structure being dissected from the surgeon's viewpoint. Examples include during bronchial dissection when performing either a right or left lower lobectomy (**Fig. 1**), middle lobectomy, or left upper lobectomy (**Fig. 2**). Adhering to a strict operative principle of passing dissecting instruments around structures in front of the pulmonary artery or its branches such that the instruments hug and are kept immediately posterior to these structures can reduce the chance of causing pulmonary artery bleeding. Also, extreme care to avoid inadvertent contact with the pulmonary artery must be taken when using energy devices when dissecting in these areas.

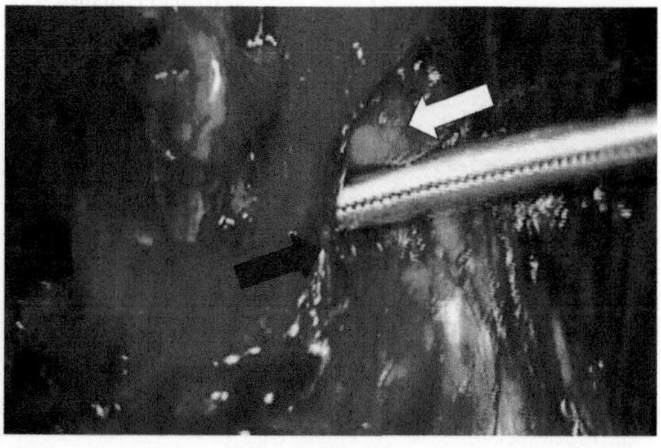

Fig. 1. Potential pulmonary artery injury during bronchial dissection as part of a VATS lower lobectomy. Passing a clamp around the bronchus (*black arrow*) can inadvertently cause injury to the pulmonary artery (*white arrow*).

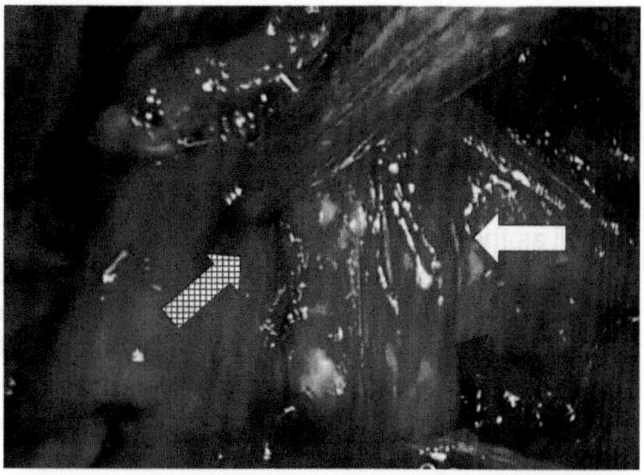

Fig. 2. Potential pulmonary artery injury during bronchial dissection as part of a VATS left upper lobectomy. Passing a clamp or stapler around the bronchus (*black arrow*) can inadvertently cause injury to the main pulmonary artery posterior to the bronchus (solid *white arrow*) or to the aspect of the pulmonary artery, which is superior to the bronchus (checked *white arrow*).

Pulmonary artery injuries that occur in these situations are not always immediately apparent. The appearance of blood during these dissection times is not necessarily uncommon and is often caused by manipulation of lymph nodes or bronchial vessels. Bleeding from these types of structures is generally not dangerous to patients but can be a nuisance that slows progress in dissection in terms of maintaining clear visualization of the desired structures. However, surgeons should never immediately assume that bleeding is from a minor structure and not a more ominous and dangerous situation, such as a pulmonary artery injury. If bleeding posterior to these structures is noted, surgeons should pause in their dissection and gently apply pressure on the anterior structure directed posteriorly for a few moments.

While holding pressure, surgeons should suction any blood from both the immediate operative vicinity as well as the entire chest. Clearing all blood from the thoracic cavity helps ensure that further bleeding will not immediately obscure the surgeons' view of the hilum. Surgeons should also note the nature of the blood. Bright red blood is more likely to be from a lymph node or bronchial vessel, particularly if it is pulsatile and high pressure. Again, this bleeding is generally not dangerous, though surgeons should take care to hold appropriate pressure and likely attempt to use cautery in the appropriate location to keep their field as clear as possible.

Dark blood that seems to gush from behind the structure that was being manipulated is a very concerning sign that some part of the adjacent pulmonary artery was injured. Surgeons should always recognize and begin to prepare for this possibility while continuing to control the situation. Both the nursing and anesthesia staff should be alerted that significant bleeding may be imminent as well as the potential need for conversion to thoracotomy for control. Surgeons should wait and not perform more surgical manipulation until the nursing staff confirms that any equipment needed for performing a thoracotomy is immediately available. Surgeons should also wait for the anesthesia staff to confirm that they have adequate monitoring and access, the ability to obtain and transfuse blood as necessary, as well as sufficient help to perform resuscitation in case sudden significant bleeding is encountered.

Holding pressure while taking the time to ensure the aforementioned measures are in place often at least temporarily stops or significantly slows any sign of bleeding. Surgeons should then carefully resume dissection. If dark bleeding is again encountered, surgeons should assume that a pulmonary artery injury has occurred. If this is the case, surgeons must plan for a method of controlling the pulmonary artery proximal to the suspected injured area. This control can be accomplished either via VATS or via conversion to thoracotomy and is discussed.

Continuing to attempt to dissect the pulmonary structure is generally not advised for 2 reasons. One, continued passage of both instruments as well as a stapler to divide the structure can lead to further or more significant injury that could be harder to both control and repair. In addition, the hilar structure anterior to the pulmonary artery in the area of the suspected injury is by itself allowing pressure to be placed on the pulmonary artery without direct manipulation. Even if surgeons can finish dissection and division of the structure without observing any more bleeding, they must continue to assume that an injury exists and be ready to deal with the situation. In particular, surgeons must be especially vigilant when a stapler has been passed and fired. Bleeding that initially seemed mild can suddenly seem significant or even torrential once the anterior structure that has been divided is no longer acting as a natural agent of tamponade. For example, as shown in **Fig. 3**, the pulmonary artery is immediately behind the lower lobe bronchus. Dividing the bronchus if a pulmonary artery injury is present can lead to sudden dramatic bleeding that can be difficult to control. In general, surgeons should temporarily leave the stapler in place to evaluate for bleeding whenever they are used to divide a structure. The stapler can be used to potentially tamponade a site of bleeding until another more appropriate instrument can be brought into the chest or a thoracotomy is performed.[20]

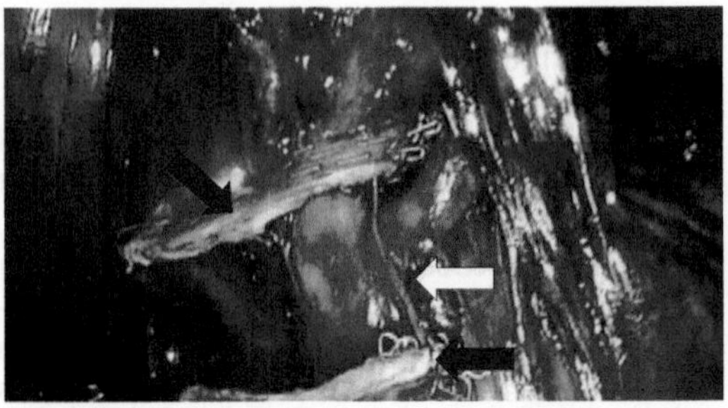

Fig. 3. Proximity of the lower lobe pulmonary artery branches in relationship to the lower lobe bronchus. After division of the lower lobe bronchus (*black arrows*), the lower lobe pulmonary artery branches are immediately and easily visualized (*white arrow*).

During Pulmonary Artery Dissection

Injury to the pulmonary artery when the pulmonary artery itself is being dissected, manipulated, or retracted can lead to a more unstable situation than that described earlier for when the pulmonary artery is injured while surgeons are working on another structure. The reason for the potentially more dangerous situation is because surgeons have typically already divided and cleared out other adjacent structures and are viewing and working on the pulmonary artery directly (**Fig. 4**). Significant blood loss can occur quickly, as there are no lung structures present that will necessarily help slow the bleeding down. Any injury in this environment must also be controlled by direct pressure to the area of injury, and surgeons must be especially careful to maintain enough pressure to tamponade the bleeding but avoid further injury

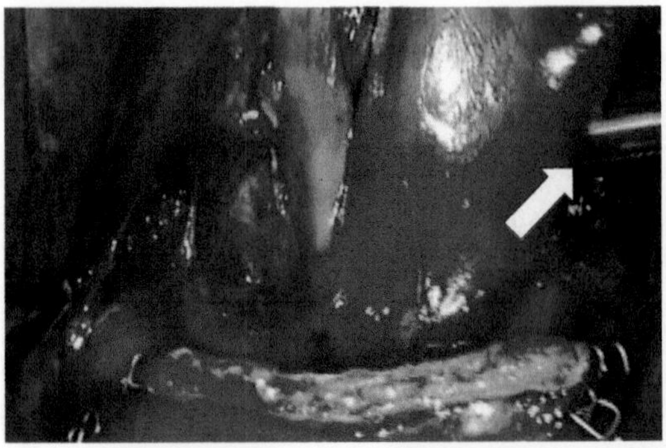

Fig. 4. Dissection of the right lower lobe pulmonary artery. Injury to the artery can occur during the passing of a dissecting instrument (*white arrow*). It also must be emphasized that excessive force during retraction can cause tearing of the vessel.

to the pulmonary artery. A tonsil sponge is particularly useful for this because it applies specific broad pressure and fits easily into a utility port sometimes easier than a sponge wrapped on a ringed clamp.

Pulmonary artery injuries in this situation can occur for a few reasons. One reason is that surgeons may be working on one area of the pulmonary artery but cause injury to another area because they did not notice that they are inadvertently causing stress. Retraction to expose the pulmonary artery can lead to excessive tension that puts the structure at risk for tearing with even gentle manipulation.[28] Bleeding in this situation can occur quite suddenly, and surgeons must always bear this in mind and be ready to control bleeding that appears. A second cause of bleeding can be an injury to, from the surgeons' viewpoint, the posterior aspect of the pulmonary artery (see **Fig. 4**). As described earlier, bleeding that seemed mild can suddenly seem quite significant if further dissection or stapler passage exacerbates a pulmonary artery injury.[29] As described earlier, surgeons must be cognizant of the possibility of sudden worsening bleeding in this situation and should again ensure all staff in the operating room are aware of the potential for bleeding and have all resources that could be necessary for obtaining control and achieving repair.

When manipulating the pulmonary artery, surgeons should be cognizant that injury to a pulmonary artery branch at the origin off the main pulmonary artery can be a more difficult situation than injury to the pulmonary artery branch more distal as it enters the lobe being removed. A more proximal injury can result in a higher volume of blood loss but, more importantly, has significant implications regarding the complexity of achieving resection and performing repair. When dissecting a pulmonary artery branch, dissection directly in the crotch of the vessel should generally be limited and more manipulation of the structure should be done on its more distal aspect as it goes toward the lung parenchyma (**Fig. 5**). Simply dividing the pulmonary artery branch, as would be done for the lobectomy anyway, generally controls injuries distal on the pulmonary artery branch. Injury to the distal aspect of the vessel is likely to have less bleeding, be easier to control, be more likely to be controlled without conversion to thoracotomy, and also has a lower chance of requiring a larger-than-planned resection, such as pneumonectomy. Injuries that involve the main pulmonary artery itself have a risk of extending more proximal. Repair will likely be more complex, and surgeons must be careful not to allow the situation to progress to uncontrolled hemorrhage, to a point where repair of the pulmonary artery injury extensively narrows the vessel or to a point where pneumonectomy is necessary to control the situation.[30]

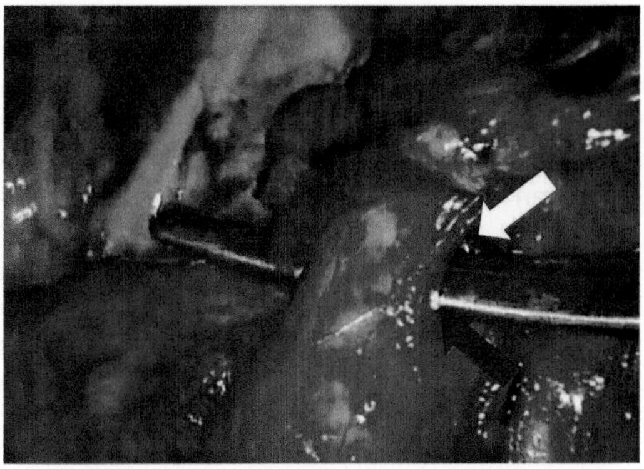

Fig. 5. Clamp being passed around the truncus pulmonary artery branch during a left upper lobectomy. Care should be taken to avoid dissection of this vessel at its origin off of the ongoing pulmonary artery (*black arrow*). Rather, dissection should be performed more distal on the vessel as it approaches the lung parenchyma (*white arrow*).

PLANNING

As with most surgical procedures, maintaining an awareness of possible complications is generally a very effective method to prevent them from occurring; disasters are easier to avoid than manage. Regardless of experience, surgeons must always be as prepared as possible for situations that may increase the risk of a pulmonary artery injury. Preoperative computer tomography (CT) scans should be carefully assessed, paying careful attention to the location of the tumor in relation to major pulmonary artery branches as well as to the appearance of lymph node abnormalities in the hilum. Factors that have been associated with the need for conversion from VATS to thoracotomy are clinical nodal disease and the presence of significant calcification on preoperative CT scan.[10,24] Another potentially preoperative method that can be helpful to surgeons in planning their operation is to use 3-dimensional reconstruction of CT angiograms, which are very effective in identifying the pulmonary artery branching patterns.[31] If surgeons anticipate based on their preoperative assessment that pulmonary artery dissection may be difficult, consideration should be given for obtaining proximal control by passing a tourniquet around the main pulmonary artery, as described later, before even attempting to manipulate the lobar pulmonary artery branches. Finally, surgeons should develop a preoperative plan for conversion with every case.

Surgeons should also recognize the role equipment available to them can play in both leading to and avoiding pulmonary artery injuries. When operating, optimizing exposure by using angled or flexible thoracoscopes and correct port placement can improve visualization and help avoid inadvertent pulmonary artery complications.[20] For example, a 30° thoracoscope can provide a range of views not possible even during an open procedure.[20] Many types of energy devices are also available and can make dissection and control of tissue and vascular structures technically easier but as described must be used very carefully to not inadvertently cause heat injury to a structure that has not yet been controlled. Clip application for delicate pulmonary artery branches should also be used only cautiously because erratic application forces can tear the vessels or later tissue manipulation can avulse the clips.[20] In addition, closing a stapler onto a clip may interfere with adequate staple application or cause significant tearing injury if the clip is dragged through tissues by the stapler knife advancing during firing.

Although stapling devices greatly facilitate the ability to perform a VATS lobectomy, continuous recognition of stapler limitations must always be maintained. Linear staplers do not pass around tubular structures in the same manner as angled instruments. Therefore, passing a dissecting instrument around a structure does not necessarily mean it will be easily divided with a stapler. Techniques to overcome difficulty in passing a stapler behind a structure include using staplers that have a curved tip or securing a red rubber catheter to the anvil of the stapler that serves to guide the stapler around pulmonary vessels.[20] Surgeons must always exercise extreme care when passing staplers around any of the hilar structures and always avoid forced manipulation. When a stapler will not easily pass around the desired structure, surgeons should consider attempting to pass the stapler from an alternative or additionally placed port. Additionally, surgeons must also keep in mind that a vascular structure can tear during the firing of a stapler when tension is causing the vessel to be stretched. Therefore, surgeons must train themselves as well as their assistants to always adjust their force of retraction when a stapler is fired so that tension on the pulmonary artery is minimized.

INTRAOPERATIVE TECHNIQUES TO CONTROL INJURY

Surgeons should avoid panic if a pulmonary artery injury occurs during a VATS lobectomy. Control of the bleeding should be obtained before considering the mechanism of repair.[32] The first step is to apply pressure with a sponge stick or similar instrument to the bleeding site. Pressure can be held directly on the bleeding site itself, on an adjacent hilar structure, or even on parenchymal lung tissue. Placing topical hemostatic agents on the site where pressure is being held can sometimes help slow or stop the bleeding. If the bleeding does stop with pressure or application of a topical hemostatic agent, generally it is advisable to not immediately resume dissection of the injured structure but rather proceed to a different step of the operation if possible. Other options include opening of the fissure to approach the pulmonary artery from another angle as well as opening the pericardium to place tape or a clamp. Clamping the pulmonary artery at the site of bleeding can extend the injury and should be avoided. As described earlier, surgeons should continuously try to keep the field as clear as possible so that bleeding does not immediately obscure their vision of the area of injury.

When a pulmonary artery injury occurs, surgeons should carefully consider their experience when choosing the most appropriate method to manage the situation. Several series have shown that the need for conversion to thoracotomy during VATS lobectomy decreases with time and experience, suggesting that surgeons gain confidence and skills to deal with difficult or unexpected situations as their overall experience increases.[23,28,33] Although pulmonary artery bleeding can be controlled and repaired by thoracoscopic techniques, it should be noted that most (92%) of a panel of 50 international experts across 16 countries on VATS lobectomy recommend conversion to open thoracotomy when major bleeding is encountered.[21] When considering attempts to control pulmonary artery bleeding thoracoscopically, surgeons should evaluate their own experience, as this same panel of experts agreed that a surgeon must have performed at least 50 cases overall and at least 20 annually to consider themselves technically proficient.[21]

One difficulty in fixing a pulmonary artery injury via VATS is that compression through the VATS incisions can effectively tamponade and control bleeding but may also obscure adequate visualization and preclude repair. Achieving proximal control of the main pulmonary artery with a clamp can be done via VATS, but the presence of the clamp can generally prevent further progress in fixing the injury. If proximal control during VATS is desired, the optimal method is likely to pass a vessel loop or suture twice around the left or right main pulmonary artery.[34] Gently applying tension to the looped suture when using this technique will allow good control while still allowing further dissection and exploration with the VATS approach, though surgeons must carefully choose the type of suture and avoid excessive tension to not saw through the main pulmonary artery. Although systemic heparinization can be considered when the artery has been clamped, this anticoagulation is likely not necessary if the period of reduced flow is kept less than 10 minutes.

As an alternative to gaining proximal control, another technique that has been described is to use a relatively thin suction device to compress the vessel in the area of injury to allow visualization that facilitates suture repair.[35] After obtaining control with either of these techniques, the pulmonary artery injury should be carefully inspected. Many injuries can be primarily repaired with the application of a permanent monofilament suture. As described earlier, surgeons should carefully evaluate their own experience when deciding if they are comfortable with doing this suturing through the VATS approach. Clips can be used to secure the knot of the suture if there is difficulty in tying the knot via VATS with a knot pusher.[20] However, as discussed earlier, surgeons should be wary of placing clips if they anticipate still needing to use a stapler to divide any remaining hilar structures in the area. When repairing the artery, surgeons should be cognizant of not causing excessive narrowing of the vessel that could put the artery at risk for immediate or delayed thrombosis.[30]

The location of injury should be taken into account when planning the repair. Pulmonary artery injuries during lower lobectomies generally do not involve the proximal pulmonary artery. Although bleeding can still be significant, attempting repair in these situations likely has less chance of causing any injury that will require division of the main pulmonary artery and, therefore, necessitating pneumonectomy for control. Conversely, pulmonary artery injuries during upper lobectomies are typically relatively close to the main pulmonary artery. Exacerbating a pulmonary artery injury in this area is more likely to lead to either an uncontrollable situation or require a pneumonectomy for control.

In general, surgeons should avoid any excessive delays in converting to a thoracotomy if necessary.[20,21] Although surgeons may develop more comfort with bleeding as their experience increases, it is always better to have opened too early rather than too late. Depending on the situation, conversion to thoracotomy can be accomplished with either using a posterior lateral thoracotomy or by enlarging the anterior access incision.[36] If the bleeding is well controlled and surgeons have not yet divided any hilar structures, using a standard thoracotomy approach may be most appropriate. If the chest must be opened more quickly to ensure adequate bleeding control, then extending the access incision is a safer option. Once the chest is opened, surgeons can use the measures described earlier to control and fix the injury. If the situation is unstable or if bleeding is uncontrolled, surgeons should manually compress the hilum and allow the patients and the situation to be stabilized. Anesthesia should be given time to catch up on volume loss before any moves are made that could result in further blood loss. If surgeons are unable to safely dissect, isolate, and control the main pulmonary artery, the entire hilum can be clamped to allow control, visualization, and repair of the pulmonary artery. In these circumstances, surgeons can consider passing a relatively straight instrument, such as a Chitwood DeBakey clamp (Scanlan International, Inc., One Scanlan Plaza, Saint Paul, MN, USA), through the original camera port so that control is achieved without impairing visualization or the ability to achieve any necessary repair.

A pulmonary artery injury should certainly be viewed as a dangerous situation. The possibility of pulmonary artery bleeding during either a VATS or an open approach should never be viewed lightly. These situations have the potential to progress to intraoperative catastrophe, and these types of incidences are likely underreported across the spectrum of surgeons. However, experienced VATS surgeons have shown that pulmonary artery bleeding can be managed safely with appropriate planning and intraoperative judgment. Reviews from several series demonstrated that intraoperative pulmonary artery bleeding during VATS leads to longer operative times and higher blood loss but is not associated with longer hospitalizations, morbidity rates, or compromised long-term outcomes.[32,33,36] These findings do not imply that the risk of a pulmonary artery injury is not significant but rather that the situation can be adequately managed and controlled with good surgical judgment.

SUMMARY

VATS lobectomy is safe overall and has many advantages for patients over an approach with a thoracotomy. With appropriate planning and operative technique, the risk of pulmonary artery injury and bleeding can be minimized. However, the risk cannot be completely eliminated; surgeons should always ensure that they are prepared to manage this situation if it occurs. Pulmonary artery injuries can be repaired via VATS, but surgeons should not hesitate to use conversion to thoracotomy when needed and depending on their VATS experience. Although pulmonary artery bleeding can potentially lead to intraoperative disasters, appropriate judgment, management, and control can avoid any impact on either short-term or long-term patient outcomes.

REFERENCES

1. Kirby TJ, Mack MJ, Landreneau RJ, et al. Initial experience with video-assisted thoracoscopic lobectomy. Ann Thorac Surg 1993;56:1248–52.
2. Swanson SJ, Herndon JE 2nd, D'Amico TA, et al. Video-assisted thoracic surgery lobectomy: report of CALGB 39802–a prospective, multi-institution feasibility study. J Clin Oncol 2007;25:4993–7.
3. Onaitis MW, Petersen RP, Balderson SS, et al. Thoracoscopic lobectomy is a safe and versatile procedure: experience with 500 consecutive patients. Ann Surg 2006;244:420–5.
4. McKenna RJ Jr, Houck W, Fuller CB. Video-assisted thoracic surgery lobectomy: experience with 1,100 cases. Ann Thorac Surg 2006;81:421–5.
5. Villamizar NR, Darrabie MD, Burfeind WR, et al. Thoracoscopic lobectomy is associated with lower morbidity compared with thoracotomy. J Thorac Cardiovasc Surg 2009;138:419–25.
6. Paul S, Altorki NK, Sheng S, et al. Thoracoscopic lobectomy is associated with lower morbidity than open lobectomy: a propensity-matched analysis from the STS database. J Thorac Cardiovasc Surg 2010;139:366–78.
7. Berry MF, Hanna J, Tong BC, et al. Risk factors for morbidity after lobectomy for lung cancer in elderly patients. Ann Thorac Surg 2009;88:1093–9.
8. Berry MF, Villamizar-Ortiz NR, Tong BC, et al. Pulmonary function tests do not predict pulmonary complications after thoracoscopic lobectomy. Ann Thorac Surg 2010;89:1044–51.
9. Ceppa DP, Kosinski AS, Berry MF, et al. Thoracoscopic lobectomy has increasing benefit in patients with poor pulmonary function: a Society of Thoracic Surgeons database analysis. Ann Surg 2012;256:487–93.
10. Villamizar NR, Darrabie M, Hanna J, et al. Impact of T status and N status on perioperative outcomes after thoracoscopic lobectomy for lung cancer. J Thorac Cardiovasc Surg 2013;145:514–20.
11. Berry MF, Onaitis MW, Tong BC, et al. Feasibility of hybrid thoracoscopic lobectomy and en-bloc chest wall resection. Eur J Cardiothorac Surg 2012;41:888–92.
12. Battoo A, Jahan A, Yang Z, et al. Thoracoscopic pneumonectomy: an 11-year experience. Chest 2014;146:1300–9.
13. Mahtabifard A, Fuller CB, McKenna RJ Jr. Video-assisted thoracic surgery sleeve lobectomy: a case series. Ann Thorac Surg 2008;85:S729–32.
14. Petersen RP, Pham D, Toloza EM, et al. Thoracoscopic lobectomy: a safe and effective strategy for patients receiving induction therapy for non-small cell lung cancer. Ann Thorac Surg 2006;82:214–8.
15. Boffa DJ, Kosinski AS, Paul S, et al. Lymph node evaluation by open or video-assisted approaches in 11,500 anatomic lung cancer resections. Ann Thorac Surg 2012;94:347–53.
16. Licht PB, Jørgensen OD, Ladegaard L, et al. A national study of nodal upstaging after thoracoscopic versus open lobectomy for clinical stage I lung cancer. Ann Thorac Surg 2013;96:943–9.
17. Merritt RE, Hoang CD, Shrager JB. Lymph node evaluation achieved by open lobectomy compared with thoracoscopic lobectomy for N0 lung cancer. Ann Thorac Surg 2013;96:1171–7.
18. Mathisen DJ. Is video-assisted thoracoscopic lobectomy inferior to open lobectomy oncologically? Ann Thorac Surg 2013;96:755–6.
19. Pickens A, McKenna RJ. Video-assisted thoracoscopic pulmonary resections. In: Kaiser LR, Kron IL, Spray TL, editors. Master of cardiothoracic surgery. 2nd edition. Philadelphia: Lippincott Williams & Wilkins; 2007. p. 92.
20. Demmy TL, James TA, Swanson SJ, et al. Troubleshooting video-assisted thoracic surgery lobectomy. Ann Thorac Surg 2005;79:1744–52.
21. Yan TD, Cao C, D'Amico TA, et al. Video-assisted thoracoscopic surgery lobectomy at 20 years: a consensus statement. Eur J Cardiothorac Surg 2014;45:633–9.
22. Roviaro G, Varoli F, Vergani C, et al. Video-assisted thoracoscopic major pulmonary resections: technical aspects, personal series of 259 patients, and review of the literature. Surg Endosc 2004;18:1551–8.
23. Puri V, Patel A, Majumder K, et al. Intraoperative conversion from video-assisted thoracoscopic surgery lobectomy to open thoracotomy: a study of causes and implications. J Thorac Cardiovasc Surg 2015;149:55–62.
24. Stephens N, Rice D, Correa A, et al. Thoracoscopic lobectomy is associated with improved short-term and equivalent oncological outcomes compared with open lobectomy for clinical stage I non-small-cell lung cancer: a propensity-matched analysis of 963 cases. Eur J Cardiothorac Surg 2014;46:607–13.
25. Liang C, Wen H, Guo Y, et al. Severe intraoperative complications during VATS lobectomy compared with thoracotomy lobectomy for early stage non-small cell lung cancer. J Thorac Dis 2013;5:513–7.
26. Samson P, Guitron J, Reed MF, et al. Predictors of conversion to thoracotomy for video-assisted thoracoscopic lobectomy: a retrospective analysis and the influence of computed tomography-based calcification assessment. J Thorac Cardiovasc Surg 2013;145:1512–8.

27. Nicastri DG, Wisnivesky JP, Litle VR, et al. Thoracoscopic lobectomy: report on safety, discharge independence, pain, and chemotherapy tolerance. J Thorac Cardiovasc Surg 2008;135:642–7.
28. Kawachi R, Tsukada H, Nakazato Y, et al. Morbidity in video-assisted thoracoscopic lobectomy for clinical stage I non-small cell lung cancer: is VATS lobectomy really safe? Thorac Cardiovasc Surg 2009;57:156–9.
29. Dunning J, Walker WS. Pulmonary artery bleeding caused during VATS lobectomy. Ann Cardiothorac Surg 2012;1:109–10.
30. Flores RM, Ihekweazu U, Dycoco J, et al. Video-assisted thoracoscopic surgery (VATS) lobectomy: catastrophic intraoperative complications. J Thorac Cardiovasc Surg 2011;142:1412–7.
31. Fukuhara K, Akashi A, Nakane S, et al. Preoperative assessment of the pulmonary artery by three-dimensional computed tomography before video-assisted thoracic surgery lobectomy. Eur J Cardiothorac Surg 2008;34:875–7.
32. Sawada S, Komori E, Yamashita M. Evaluation of video-assisted thoracoscopic surgery lobectomy requiring emergency conversion to thoracotomy. Eur J Cardiothorac Surg 2009;36:487–90.
33. Jones RO, Casali G, Walker WS. Does failed video-assisted lobectomy for lung cancer prejudice immediate and long-term outcomes? Ann Thorac Surg 2008;86:235–9.
34. Watanabe A, Koyanagi T, Nakashima S, et al. How to clamp the main pulmonary artery during video-assisted thoracoscopic surgery lobectomy. Eur J Cardiothorac Surg 2007;31:129–31.
35. Mei J, Pu Q, Liao H, et al. A novel method for troubleshooting vascular injury during anatomic thoracoscopic pulmonary resection without conversion to thoracotomy. Surg Endosc 2013;27(2):530–7.
36. Yamashita S, Tokuishi K, Moroga T, et al. Totally thoracoscopic surgery and troubleshooting for bleeding in non-small cell lung cancer. Ann Thorac Surg 2013;95:994–9.

Intraoperative Tracheal Injury

Natalie Lui, MD, Cameron Wright, MD*

KEYWORDS

• Tracheal injury • Tracheal repair • Esophagectomy complications
• Percutaneous tracheostomy complications

KEY POINTS

- Intraoperative tracheal injury, a rare but devastating complication, is estimated to have an incidence of 0.4% during transhiatal esophagectomy at high-volume centers, 0.005% during single-lumen intubation, 0.05% during double-lumen intubation, and 0.2% during percutaneous dilatational tracheostomy.
- Prevention by careful case selection is key: transhiatal esophagectomy should be avoided in patients with proximal esophageal tumors who underwent neoadjuvant therapy, and percutaneous tracheostomy should be avoided in patients with short, thick necks.
- Early recognition leads to improved outcomes. Patients present with a sudden loss in airway pressure, air leaking into the operative field, or mediastinal and subcutaneous emphysema.
- Treatment starts with airway control. An existing single-lumen endotracheal tube may be advanced beyond the injury, or it can be advanced into the left main bronchus in preparation for single-lung ventilation during a right thoracotomy.
- Primary buttressed repair using interrupted absorbable suture and an intercostal muscle flap is recommended, through either a left cervical incision for proximal injuries or a right thoracotomy for distal injuries.
- Conservative management has been used safely in select patients with superficial injuries caused by intubation or tracheostomy who have adequate ventilation and nonprogressive mediastinal or subcutaneous emphysema.

INTRODUCTION

Intraoperative tracheal injury is a rare but potentially devastating complication. The most common procedures associated with tracheal injury are esophagectomy, endotracheal intubation, and tracheostomy. Literature on this topic contains only case series and case reports. They show trends in prevention, diagnosis, and management that can prepare clinicians should they encounter this complication.

PREVENTION

The importance of prevention cannot be overstated. For esophagectomy, proper case selection is paramount. Patients with tumors in the upper or middle third of the esophagus, especially those who have undergone neoadjuvant radiation, are at higher risk of tracheal injury. Careful esophageal dissection and mediastinal lymphadenectomy is also essential. A transthoracic approach should be used if there is any concern for tracheobronchial involvement.

For tracheostomy, an open instead of percutaneous approach should be used in patients with short, thick necks. Bronchoscopic guidance can assist in prevention and early recognition of tracheal injuries. Difficult tracheostomy and intubation should be performed by experienced teams to avoid multiple attempts.

The authors have nothing to disclose.
Division of Thoracic Surgery, Massachusetts General Hospital, 55 Fruit Street, Blake 1570, Boston, MA 02114, USA
* Corresponding author.
E-mail address: cdwright@partners.org

Thorac Surg Clin 25 (2015) 249–254
http://dx.doi.org/10.1016/j.thorsurg.2015.04.008
1547-4127/15/$ – see front matter

DIAGNOSIS

Early recognition of tracheal injury is important for good outcomes. The method and extent of injury determine the patient's signs and symptoms. Small injuries that are not recognized may heal on their own, although some lead to tracheal stenosis or fistula.

Tracheal injury during esophagectomy is usually recognized immediately. Often the injury is visible within the operative field. Unrecognized injuries may arise from thermal injury or injury to the left mainstem bronchus where dissection of the subcarinal lymph nodes takes place. Sudden loss of airway pressures and air leaking from the incision are also common. More rarely, pneumothorax, even tension pneumothorax, may be the presenting sign. Even pneumoperitoneum and tension pneumoperitoneum have been reported.[1,2] A delay in diagnosis can occur when pneumoperitoneum is the only sign.[3] Postoperatively, persistent air leak and/or subcutaneous or mediastinal emphysema should cause concern for tracheal injury.

Hulscher and colleagues[4] described six patients with tracheal injury during esophagectomy. The injury was recognized intraoperatively in five patients, and on postoperative Day one in the remaining patient. The latter patient self-extubated and after reintubation, air was leaking from the cervical incision. Bartels and colleagues[5] described 31 tracheobronchial injuries that were discovered postoperatively after esophagectomy. The patients presented with pneumomediastinum (eight), pneumothorax (19), or a fistula between the trachea and esophageal remnant or conduit (four).

When tracheal injury occurs during endotracheal intubation, there may be no immediate signs. Massard and coworkers[3] described eight patients who were diagnosed postoperatively, from 6 to 126 hours after their operations. All of them developed mediastinal and subcutaneous emphysema, and two patients had a pneumothorax. Imaging studies may show subtle signs of tracheal injury. Deviation of the tip of the endotracheal tube, especially to the right, on chest radiograph, or a large endotracheal tube cuff diameter on computed tomography, should raise concern.

METHODS OF INJURY

Esophagectomy

Intraoperative tracheal injury has been reported in transabdominal and transthoracic mediastinal dissection. The cause may be traction or thermal injury during either esophageal dissection or mediastinal lymphadenectomy. The trachea is at highest risk during the blunt mediastinal dissection of a transhiatal esophagectomy. The posterior membranous wall is most commonly injured. As described previously, careful case selection is key.

Large case series have shown a low incidence of tracheal injury during esophagectomy. Orringer and colleagues[6] described 2029 patients who underwent transhiatal esophagectomy. Eight (0.4%) patients had intraoperative membranous tracheobronchial tears. Four patients were repaired through a right thoracotomy, and four patients through a partial sternotomy. The authors warned against attempting transhiatal esophagectomy in patients with cancers that invade the tracheobronchial tree. Yannopoulos and colleagues[7] described 750 patients who underwent transhiatal esophagectomy. Three (0.4%) patients had intraoperative tracheal injury. One patient was repaired through a median sternotomy, and two patients through the planned cervical incision. Luketich and colleagues[8] described 1033 patients who underwent minimally invasive esophagectomy, and there were no tracheal injuries reported.

Several case series showed trends in tracheal injury during esophagectomy. Koshenkov and colleagues[9] described 425 patients who underwent esophagectomy, of which 88% were transhiatal esophagectomies. Seven (1.6%) patients had intraoperative tracheobronchial injuries. Patients with these injuries were older, more likely to have proximal tumors and squamous cell carcinoma, and more likely to have undergone neoadjuvant chemoradiation. Prompt recognition was important in outcome. Perioperative death occurred in none of the three patients whose injuries were identified intraoperatively, and three of the four patients whose injuries were detected postoperatively.

Hulscher and colleagues[4] described 383 patients who underwent esophagectomy. Six (1.6%) patients had tracheal injuries, five during transhiatal dissections and one during a transthoracic dissection. These patients were more likely to have pulmonary complications, such as pneumonia or atelectasis, compared with patients without tracheal injury. They also had longer ventilation times and intensive care unit stays.

Bartels and colleagues[5] described 785 patients who underwent esophagectomy for malignancy. Two (0.3%) had intraoperative tracheal injuries that were recognized during the operation and repaired primarily, and 31 (3.9%) had tracheobronchial injuries discovered on postoperative Days 1 to 30. Based on the timing and location of these injuries, they were attributed to intraoperative injury not recognized during the operation (four), cuff pressure from the tracheostomy tube in the setting of prolonged respiratory failure (two), peritracheal inflammation caused by an insufficiently drained cervical anastomotic leak (seven), or ischemia caused by extensive peritracheal dissection (18). Risk factors for tracheobronchial injury included neoadjuvant chemoradiation for tumors at or above the carina and transthoracic en bloc resection with extended mediastinal lymphadenopathy.

Tracheostomy

Tracheal injury can occur during percutaneous and open tracheostomy. A frequent cause is the guidewire or dilator used in percutaneous dilatational tracheostomy. The injury is often in the posterior membranous wall.

Kumar and colleagues[10] described 345 patients who underwent percutaneous dilatational tracheostomy and postprocedure chest radiograph. Ninety-three (27%) patients had an adverse event during the procedure. These included 34 tracheal ring fractures, eight minor (single puncture) posterior tracheal wall injuries, and one major (mucosal tear) posterior tracheal wall injury.

Simon and colleagues[11] reported 71 cases of death caused by complications of percutaneous dilatational tracheostomy. The estimated incidence is 0.17%. Of these, 15% were caused by tracheal injury. Factors involved in these cases were performing the procedure without bronchoscopy (five), an inexperienced procedural team (four), an obese patient (one), a child (one), kinking of the guidewire (two), and spine abnormalities (one). Thus a kinked guidewire should raise concern of tracheal injury.

Berrouschot and colleagues[12] described 71 patients who underwent percutaneous dilatational tracheostomy, with and without bronchoscopic guidance. Three (4.2%) patients had tracheal injuries. One patient died of a tension pneumothorax, and the other two patients underwent right thoracotomy and primary repair. All three patients did not have bronchoscopic monitoring during the tracheostomy, and the injuries were thought to be caused by steep insertion of the dilators.

Almost complete tracheal transection has been reported after difficult percutaneous dilatational tracheostomy.[13] Tracheal injury has also been reported in tracheostomy tube change.[1]

Intubation

The incidence of intraoperative tracheal injury caused by intubation is unknown but estimated at 0.005% for single-lumen intubations and 0.05% for double-lumen intubations.[14] These injuries can be caused by the tip of the endotracheal tube itself during insertion or overinflation of the cuff. They often involve a longitudinal laceration of the posterior membranous trachea (**Fig. 1**).

Massard and colleagues[3] described 14 patients with tracheal injury, including nine patients after single-lumen intubation and one patient after double-lumen intubation. All nine patients who had single-lumen intubation were short women, with heights ranging from 148 to 165 cm. The injuries were located in the upper (one), middle (one), and lower (seven) third of the trachea; and on the right (eight) and middle (one) of the membranosa. Five injuries extended to the right mainstem bronchus. Because of the predominance of injuries in the distal right trachea, the authors hypothesized that the most common mechanism of injury is overinflation of the endotracheal tube cuff. They posited that after a right mainstem intubation, the cuff is inflated in the larger carinal space, then the endotracheal tube is withdrawn without adequately deflation. It may be easier to insert an endotracheal tube into the right mainstem in a short patient, and easier to overinflate a cuff in a woman with a narrower trachea.

Schneider and colleagues[14] described 16 patients with tracheal injury after intubation, 14 patients after single-lumen intubation and two patients after double-lumen. All injuries were longitudinal lacerations in the membranous trachea, or a carinal perforation leading to a longitudinal laceration of a main bronchus. The median length of

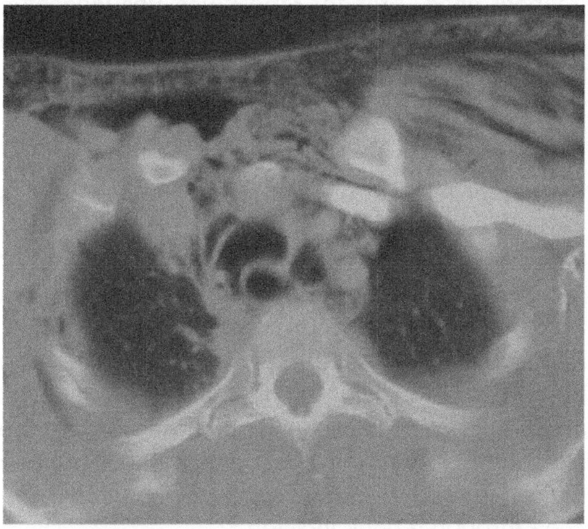

Fig. 1. Computed tomographic image of a posterior tracheal injury caused by emergent endotracheal intubation in a patient with a chronic obstructive pulmonary disease flare, with resulting pneumomediastinum and subcutaneous emphysema. The patient underwent repair through a transverse cervical incision and partial sternotomy. The tear was repaired by a longitudinal tracheotomy over the posterior tear.

injury was 4 cm. Ten of the cases were emergent intubations. The authors thought that multiple vigorous attempts at intubation by an inexperienced anesthesiologist and the inappropriate use of a stylet were additional risk factors.

Other

There have been a few case reports of tracheal injury caused by median sternotomy.[15–17] In all cases, there was clear air leaking from the operative field immediately after sternotomy. In two cases, the endotracheal tube cuff was damaged, and the endotracheal tube was exchanged and advanced beyond the injury. In one case, there was a 6-mm laceration on the anterior trachea between the second and third tracheal rings.[17] In another case, there was a 10-mm laceration at the sixth and seventh tracheal rings.[16] Primary repair was completed in all cases. The operation was completed as planned[15] or postponed for a week[16] without further complications.

Lemaire and colleagues[18] described 2145 patients who underwent mediastinoscopy. Only two (0.09%) patients had tracheal injury. Hammoud and colleagues[19] described 2137 patients who underwent mediastinoscopy, and no tracheal injuries were noted.

Kouerinis and colleagues[20] described a case where the membranous trachea was injured during resection of a locally advanced lung cancer that had invaded the mediastinum but not the trachea itself. They discovered a 3-cm longitudinal laceration in the membranous wall near the tracheal rings. Primary repair was unsuccessful, so they placed an intercostal muscle flap between the trachea and esophagus.

REPAIR

Repair of intraoperative tracheal injuries begins with airway control. Strategies depend on the location of the injury and the planned access for repair. The site of injury can be packed tightly so that the patient can be ventilated temporarily. Proximal tracheal injuries may be repaired through a left cervical incision or partial sternotomy. The single-lumen endotracheal tube may simply be advanced beyond the injury. The anterior trachea may need to be divided to access the posterior trachea through a neck incision.[21]

Distal tracheal injuries should be repaired through a right thoracotomy. The single-lumen endotracheal tube may be advanced past the injury into the left mainstem bronchus or exchanged for a double-lumen tube. Great caution should be used if a double-lumen tube is deemed necessary so as to not worsen the injury. Bronchoscopic guidance is prudent in that case. If the patient does not tolerate single-lung ventilation, but extensive injury precludes the use of a tracheal cuff, then the right and left mainstem bronchi may be intubated separately with pediatric endotracheal tubes.[22]

During transhiatal esophagectomy, there is no access to the trachea through the abdominal incision. The patient must be turned to the left lateral decubitus position for a right thoracotomy. If the injury occurs during the cervical dissection, it may be repaired through the preexisting cervical incision or may require partial sternotomy.

After tracheal injuries during open or percutaneous tracheostomy, exposure of the lateral trachea or posterior trachea is difficult. Anterior tracheal transverse division or longitudinal incision may be required to access the injury. More distally in the neck, the lateral trachea is more accessible and division is usually not necessary.

Primary buttressed repair using intercostal muscle and interrupted absorbable suture, such as 4-O Vicryl or 4-0 PDS, should be used. Devitalized tissue should be debrided, but this is rare if the injury is recognized early. Extensive dissection around the trachea should be avoided so the vascular supply remains intact. Careful avoidance of injuring the recurrent laryngeal nerve is also important.

Buttressed repair is important. Case reports describe tracheal repair reinforced with gastric conduit,[4] pericardial patch,[23] sternocleidomastoid muscle,[2] and cyanoacrylate glue.[24] One case report describes reinforcement with Gore-Tex, which required removal because of infection 22 months later.[25]

After the repair, the endotracheal tube should be moved enough to confirm it has not been sewn in place. An air leak test can be performed by filling the field with saline and slowly increasing ventilatory pressure. Bronchoscopy should usually be performed to ensure the integrity of the repair. At this point, the esophagectomy (if performed) may be completed with a thoracic or cervical anastomosis.

Conservative Management

There has been a trend toward nonoperative management in cases with superficial injury caused by intubation or tracheostomy, especially if they are recognized postoperatively. However, nonoperative management must be used with caution, because delayed surgical repair may lead to more tissue loss, mediastinal infection, and poor healing.

Schneider and colleagues[14] described 29 patients with tracheal injury after intubation or

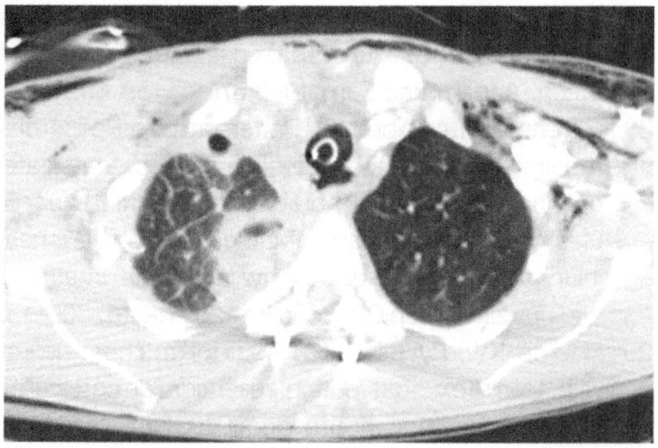

Fig. 2. Computed tomographic image of a posterior tracheal injury caused by percutaneous tracheostomy. The patient underwent percutaneous tracheostomy and subsequently developed a right pneumothorax and subcutaneous emphysema. Bronchoscopy showed a 4-cm defect of the posterior tracheal membrane starting just distal to the cricoid. The tracheal injury healed with nonoperative management by placement of an extra-long tracheosotmy tube distal to the injury site.

tracheostomy. Eleven were treated nonoperatively. The criteria they used to determine that nonoperative management were superficial injuries or injuries covered by the esophagus, adequate ventilation, and nonprogressive subcutaneous emphysema. Broad-spectrum antibiotics were given (**Fig. 2**). All 11 patients survived without mediastinitis or conversion to surgical repair.

Ovari and colleagues[26] described three patients who had tracheal injuries during head and neck procedures. One injury was recognized intraoperatively, and two injuries were recognized postoperatively after the development of subcutaneous emphysema. Tracheostomy with broad-spectrum antibiotics was used in all patients with injury without further complication.

SUMMARY

Intraoperative tracheal injuries are rare but potentially fatal complications. They occur most often during transhiatal esophagectomy, percutaneous dilatational tracheostomy, and endotracheal intubation. Surgeons should be prepared to diagnose and manage these injuries promptly to improve outcomes for these patients.

REFERENCES

1. Pang PY, Su JW. Tracheal injury causing massive pneumoperitoneum following change of a tracheostomy tube. Ann Acad Med Singapore 2012;41(11):532–3.
2. Lal AB, Kumar N, Sami KA. Tension pneumoperitoneum from tracheal tear during pharyngolaryngoesophagectomy. Anesth Analg 1995;80(2):408–9.
3. Massard G, Rouge C, Dabbagh A, et al. Tracheobronchial lacerations after intubation and tracheostomy. Ann Thorac Surg 1996;61(5):1483–7.
4. Hulscher JB, ter Hofstede E, Kloek J, et al. Injury to the major airways during subtotal esophagectomy: incidence, management, and sequelae. J Thorac Cardiovasc Surg 2000;120(6):1093–6.
5. Bartels HE, Stein HJ, Siewert JR. Tracheobronchial lesions following oesophagectomy: prevalence, predisposing factors and outcome. Br J Surg 1998; 85(3):403–6.
6. Orringer MB, Marshall B, Chang AC, et al. Two thousand transhiatal esophagectomies: changing trends, lessons learned. Ann Surg 2007;246(3): 363–72 [discussion: 372–4].
7. Yannopoulos P, Theodoridis P, Manes K. Esophagectomy without thoracotomy: 25 years of experience over 750 patients. Langenbecks Arch Surg 2009;394(4):611–6.
8. Luketich JD, Pennathur A, Awais O, et al. Outcomes after minimally invasive esophagectomy: review of over 1000 patients. Ann Surg 2012;256(1): 95–103.
9. Koshenkov VP, Yakoub D, Livingstone AS, et al. Tracheobronchial injury in the setting of an esophagectomy for cancer: postoperative discovery a bad omen. J Surg Oncol 2014;109(8):804–7.
10. Kumar VM, Grant CA, Hughes MW, et al. Role of routine chest radiography after percutaneous dilatational tracheostomy. Br J Anaesth 2008;100(5): 663–6.
11. Simon M, Metschke M, Braune SA, et al. Death after percutaneous dilatational tracheostomy: a systematic review and analysis of risk factors. Crit Care 2013;17(5):R258.
12. Berrouschot J, Oeken J, Steiniger L, et al. Perioperative complications of percutaneous dilational tracheostomy. Laryngoscope 1997;107(11 Pt 1): 1538–44.
13. Kedjanyi WK, Gupta D. Near total transection of the trachea following percutaneous dilatational tracheostomy. J R Coll Surg Edinb 2001;46(4):242–3.
14. Schneider T, Storz K, Dienemann H, et al. Management of iatrogenic tracheobronchial injuries: a retrospective analysis of 29 cases. Ann Thorac Surg 2007;83(6):1960–4.
15. Renna M, Gillbe C. A novel complication of sternotomy for cardiac surgery. J Cardiothorac Vasc Anesth 1994;8(1):133.
16. Takanami I. Tracheal laceration: a rare complication of median sternotomy. J Thorac Cardiovasc Surg 2001;122(1):184.
17. Raut M, Maheshwari A, Shivnani G, et al. Anterior tracheal injury during sternotomy. J Cardiothorac Vasc Anesth 2013;27(5):e60–1.

18. Lemaire A, Nikolic I, Petersen T, et al. Nine-year single center experience with cervical mediastinoscopy: complications and false negative rate. Ann Thorac Surg 2006;82(4):1185–9 [discussion: 1189–90].
19. Hammoud ZT, Anderson RC, Meyers BF, et al. The current role of mediastinoscopy in the evaluation of thoracic disease. J Thorac Cardiovasc Surg 1999; 118(5):894–9.
20. Kouerinis IA, Loutsidis AE, Hountis PA, et al. Treatment of iatrogenic injury of membranous trachea with intercostal muscle flap. Ann Thorac Surg 2004;78(5):e85–6.
21. Angelillo-Mackinlay T. Transcervical repair of distal membranous tracheal laceration. Ann Thorac Surg 1995;59(2):531–2.
22. Gitter R, Daniel TM, Kesser BW, et al. Membranous tracheobronchial injury repaired with gastric serosal patch. Ann Thorac Surg 1999;67(4):1159–60.
23. Gorenstein LA, Abel JG, Patterson GA. Pericardial repair of a tracheal laceration during transhiatal esophagectomy. Ann Thorac Surg 1992;54(4):784–6.
24. George SV, Samarasam I, Mathew G, et al. Tracheal injury during oesophagectomy: incidence, treatment and outcome. Trop Gastroenterol 2011;32(4):309–13.
25. Millikan KW, Pytynia KB. Repair of tracheal defect with Gore-Tex graft during resection of carcinoma of the esophagus. J Surg Oncol 1997;66(2):134–7.
26. Ovari A, Just T, Dommerich S, et al. Conservative management of post-intubation tracheal tears-report of three cases. J Thorac Dis 2014;6(6): E85–91.

Massive Airway Hemorrhage

Sai Yendamuri, MD[a,b,*]

KEYWORDS

• Hemoptysis • Rigid bronchoscopy • Bronchial artery embolization • Thoracic surgery

KEY POINTS

- Massive hemoptysis requires a systematic yet flexible multidisciplinary approach.
- Initial treatment consists of stabilization, securing the airway, and nonsurgical temporization of the bleeding source.
- Rigid bronchoscopy is the best way to secure an airway in patients with massive hemoptysis.
- Delayed surgery after stabilization leads to the best surgical results.

INTRODUCTION

Acute airway hemorrhage represents a challenge to the thoracic surgical team, including the surgeon as well as the anesthesiologist. Although torrential hemorrhage is rare, a stepwise approach to dealing with this catastrophic situation is necessary to salvage patients. This stepwise approach should be built on the availability of necessary infrastructure and expertise. This article examines the cause of airway hemorrhage and provides an overview of the management strategies that the surgical team should be aware of to deal with this surgical emergency.

The airway has a dead space of approximately 150 mL. The mucociliary mechanism and cough reflex can evacuate some amount of blood; but even a modest amount of bleeding can overcome these mechanisms, leading to asphyxiation. The definition of massive hemoptysis varies from 100 to 1000 mL over a 24-hour period; the intent of this quantification being the identification of patients needing immediate intervention.[1–3] However, the urgency of intervention depends on several factors, including the overall functional status of patients, rapidity of bleeding over shorter intervals of time, cause of the disease, and available treatment options. Therefore, investigators have proposed alternative definitions of life-threatening hemoptysis based on the magnitude of the functional effects of the hemoptysis rather than just the measurement of the same.[4] Some criteria suggested for such definitions include the need for hospitalization, transfusion, intubation, hypoxemia, and hypotension.[5–7] These criteria have been at least partly motivated by the practical problem of unreliable patient measurements of hemoptysis.

CAUSE

Airway hemorrhage can be broadly divided as arising from 2 sources. The first source is the proximal airways, such as that arising from the trachea, mainstem bronchi, and proximal lobar bronchi. The second is from the distal airway.

1. Proximal airway bleeding: **Box 1** lists possible sources of proximal airway bleeding. Malignant tumors of the airway are by far the most common sources of tracheobronchial bleeding. An example of one such source is shown in **Fig. 1**. The main implication of identifying proximal airway bleeding is that interventional

The author has no competing interests to declare.

[a] Department of Thoracic Surgery, Roswell Park Cancer Institute, Elm and Carlton Streets, Buffalo, NY 14263, USA; [b] Yashoda Hospitals, Alexander Road, Secunderabad, Telangana 500003, India
* Roswell Park Cancer Institute, Elm and Carlton Streets, Buffalo, NY 14263.
E-mail address: sai.yendamuri@roswellpark.org

Thorac Surg Clin 25 (2015) 255–260
http://dx.doi.org/10.1016/j.thorsurg.2015.04.009

Box 1
Causes of proximal airway bleeding

Malignant
- Squamous cell cancer
- Adenoid cystic carcinoma
- Carcinoid
- Mucoepidermoid cancer

Benign
- Iatrogenic
- Tracheo-innominate fistula
- Broncholithiasis
- Inflammatory lesions of the airway
- Dieulafoy disease of the bronchus
- Trauma

pulmonary techniques can be potentially used to arrest bleeding. Also, the proximal airway is within reach of a rigid bronchoscope, which is the instrument of choice for managing this situation in the operating room.

2. Distal airway bleeding: There are many more causes of distal airway bleeding as virtually every lung pathology can lead to some amount of bleeding. The more prominent etiologic groups are summarized in **Box 2**. The implication of this etiologic grouping is that bleeding caused by these conditions cannot always be managed by interventional pulmonary methods. Management depends on the treatment of the primary cause.

MANAGEMENT STRATEGY

The management of airway bleeding depends on a structured yet flexible approach by a multidisciplinary team of anesthesia, thoracic surgery, interventional pulmonology, and interventional radiology. One possible schema for an overall management strategy is summarized in **Fig. 2**. This strategy can be divided into 3 steps:

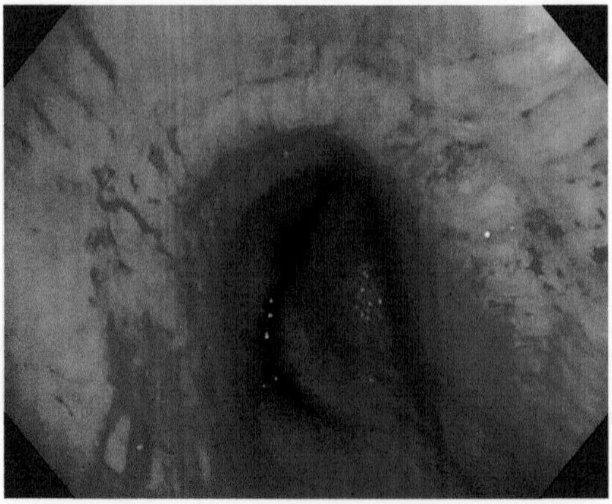

Fig. 1. Endobronchial tumor. Adenocystic carcinoma in distal trachea.

Box 2
Causes of distal airway bleeding

Vasculites

Coagulopathy

Cardiovascular diseases
- Mitral stenosis
- Arteriovenous malformations
- Pulmonary embolism

Pulmonary parenchymal diseases
- Lymphangioleiomyomatosis
- Pulmonary capillary hemangiomatosis
- Pulmonary hemosiderosis

Infections
- Bronchiectasis
- Aspergillosis
- Tuberculosis
- Lung abscess
- Bronchitis

Malignancy
- Primary lung cancer
- Metastases

Foreign body

Iatrogenic (eg, computed tomography–guided biopsy)

STABILIZATION

As in all surgical emergencies, the first step consists of assessing the stability of the airway and the circulatory system. Once this is done, a brief history and physical examination are performed. Bilateral large-bore peripheral intravenous access is obtained; in this process, investigations are sent off for regular blood work, coagulation profile and blood typing, and cross matching. A frontal chest radiograph is obtained; if patients are stable, a computed tomography scan adds invaluable information. The operating room team and the interventional team (thoracic surgeon and/or interventional pulmonologist and the interventional radiologist) are alerted. Opiates are administered judiciously to decrease forceful coughing without altering the sensorium. Any coagulopathy, if

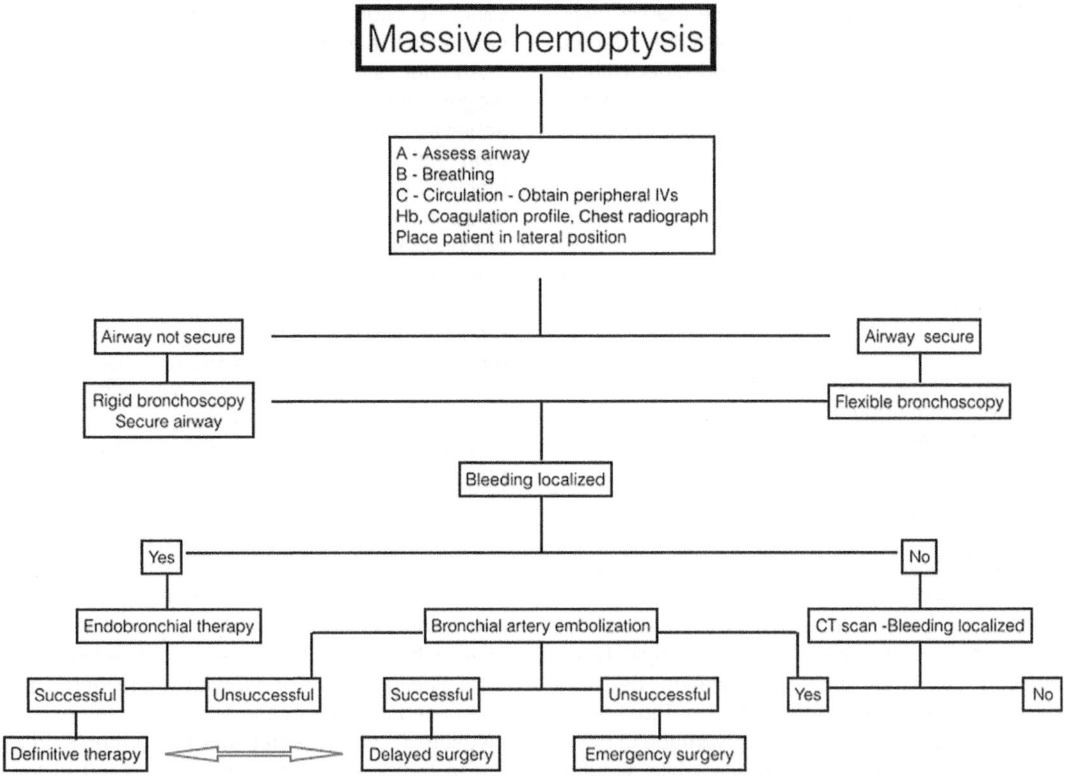

Fig. 2. Algorithm for management of massive hemoptysis. CT, computed tomography; Hb, hemoglobin; IVs, intravenous injections.

present, is corrected and blood volume repleted. Lung function often cannot be assessed by formal pulmonary function tests; but a combination of immediate history before the episode and the ability of patients to walk a reasonable distance or climb stairs suffices, drawing the conclusion that at least a lobectomy can be tolerated, if necessary. If a unilateral cause of bleeding is suspected based on the chest radiograph, patients should be laid with the affected side down. If hemoptysis is moderate, an urgent bronchoscopy is scheduled. If the hemoptysis is unrelenting, it hampers visualization as well as lateralization. If the hemoptysis has already stopped, it may be difficult to pinpoint a small source. Therefore, the most appropriate time for bronchoscopy is when the hemoptysis has almost stopped; but often, such timing is not in the hands of the bronchoscopist. If the hemoptysis is severe enough to potentially cause asphyxiation, patients are taken to the operating room to secure the airway.

SECURING THE AIRWAY

Although intubation with a double lumen tube to secure the airway sounds enticing, this strategy is beset with practical problems. Small bronchoscopes to guide double lumen tube placement do not have wide-bore suction channels and are, therefore, ineffective at providing visualization in the face of bleeding. Also, the proximal airway cannot be examined with the tube in place; therapeutic bronchoscopy cannot be performed through a double lumen tube. Given these limitations, the author recommends that initial airway be secured with the largest single lumen endotracheal tube possible. Before intubation commences, the oral cavity and hypopharynx must be quickly screened for a bleeding source. Nasotracheal intubation is discouraged because of the size of the endotracheal tube required for therapeutic bronchoscopy and the fact that a nasal single lumen tube may be difficult to advance to the mainstem bronchus to protect the airway in the face of uncontrolled bleeding. The author's preference is to intubate under bronchoscopic visualization. This practice enables the detection of proximal tracheal sources of bleeding that would not be possible with laryngoscopic intubation. If intubation and bronchoscopy demonstrate a proximal airway source of hemorrhage that is significant, a rigid bronchoscope provides the most secure airway and should be readily available. A rigid bronchoscope enables the evacuation of large amounts of blood and clots without impeding ventilation. Having a rigid bronchoscope in place enables the deployment of several therapeutic tools as discussed later.

BLEEDING CONTROL

Once the airway is secure, the next goal of the treatment team is bleeding control. The choices are

1. Flexible or rigid bronchoscopy
2. Endoluminal approaches
3. Surgery (transthoracic approaches)

Bleeding Control by Flexible/Rigid Bronchoscopy

Rigid bronchoscopy, the preferred method of bleeding control in hemoptysis, is an essential skill for the thoracic surgeon. The use of rigid bronchoscopy requires good cooperation between the anesthesiologist and the surgeon. Rigid bronchoscopy provides the distinct advantage of being able to visualize the bleeding site while simultaneously providing ventilation. Blood and blood clots can be more easily evacuated, and instrument exchanges are quick. All therapeutic modalities for bleeding control can be applied using a rigid bronchoscope. In addition, a rigid bronchoscope can be used to core out an offending tumor. Flexible bronchoscopes have become more advanced over the last 2 decades. Visualization is superb, and working channel diameters have increased to accommodate an array of devices. Often, a flexible bronchoscope is passed through a rigid bronchoscope to enhance visualization.

For small bleeding sources, cold saline lavage or dilute epinephrine may arrest bleeding. Cold saline lavage involves the repeated application of approximately 50-mL aliquots of saline on ice (4°C) until bleeding stops. Conlan and Hurwitz[8] first described this technique by rigid bronchoscopy in 1980. In the 12 patients in this series, each had at least temporary cessation of bleeding. This method is also easily applied by flexible bronchoscopy. Unfortunately, dilute epinephrine application (1:20,000) does not work as well because the drug is easily washed away with bleeding. Other agents used include oral and intravenous use of tranexamic acid that is well described in the literature. However, endobronchial application has only recently been described; therefore, the body of literature to support its use is scant.[9] Similarly, small case series have been published on various combinations of fibrin and thrombin application via the endobronchial route.[10,11]

Another strategy for bleeding control from bigger sources is by tamponade, which can be achieved through several means. The most common way of introducing a standard bronchial blocker (usually used to facilitate single lung ventilation) is through the endobronchial tube itself, under bronchoscopic guidance. Another alternative is to introduce it through the cords alongside the endotracheal tube. Even though maneuvering the tube this way is a little more cumbersome than through the tube, it leaves the endotracheal tube open for further bronchoscopic evacuation of clots and other therapies. Segmental bronchial bleeding can be stopped by tamponade with the use of a Fogarty catheter, a standard pulmonary artery catheter, or other specially designed catheters. If left in for a long time, necessary care should be taken to minimize the incidence of mucosal necrosis, such as inflating the balloon to the minimum and to deflate it periodically.[12–15] Similarly, other devices like a spigot, oxidized cellulose mesh, surgical glue (n-butyl-cyanoacrylate), and stents have been used in limited case series as a temporizing measure to stabilize patients for further therapy. These tamponading devices can be left in for a long time to facilitate more definitive therapy. However, postobstructive pneumonia may develop if left in too long.[16–20]

Definitive control of bleeding can also be obtained endobronchially using energy devices. These devices include electrocautery, cryotherapy, laser, and argon plasma coagulation. The requirements for these devices include the lesion to be endobronchially accessible and that the bleeding has slowed enough to enable therapy. These therapies are most applicable to tumors but can be used in other pathology, such as submucosal bronchial arteries. Each of these therapies are equally effective, and the choice of therapy used depends on the available tools and surgeon preference. However, each modality has some advantages and disadvantages in special situations. Electrocautery is the cheapest modality to use. Small case series show it to be effective, but a large body of data is lacking.[21] Argon plasma coagulation has the distinct advantage of working well at corners that are sometimes difficult to approach by laser. Also, a small amount of bleeding is less of an issue with this modality. Investigators have used this therapeutic approach quite effectively.[22] Laser photocoagulation has been mostly applied with Nd-YAG lasers. Lasers have a greater depth penetration and can, therefore, open up an obstructed airway more effectively while at the same time controlling bleeding.

However, this method requires a reasonably dry field for application. Effectiveness for control of hemoptysis has been reported to be between 60% and 94%.[23,24] Cryotherapy is a relatively new modality that has been used in the setting of hemoptysis. It is thought to control bleeding by induction of thrombosis in the offending lesion.[25,26] Cryotherapy has the distinct advantage of being able to remove large clots easily without requiring a reduction in the fraction of inspired oxygen of the oxygen levels used for ventilating patients.

Interventional Radiology Approaches

Bronchial artery embolization (BAE) is a very useful adjunct in the management of massive hemoptysis. It is based on the principle that most massive hemoptysis is from the high-pressure bronchial arterial circulation (>90%) and very rarely from the low-pressure pulmonary artery circulation (5%).[27] It is used after stabilization of patients and securing the airway. Bronchoscopy before the embolization is sometimes useful if the bleeding can be lateralized. The usual course of embolization is to access the femoral artery via a 3F catheter. Individual bronchial arteries are identified, and arteries suspected to be the cause of hemorrhage by radiological characteristics (tortuosity or extravasation) are embolized with microspheres, an absorbable gelatin sponge (Gelfoam, Pharmacia and Upjohn Company, Kalamazoo, MI), or coils. When patients are properly selected, BAE can control hemoptysis 90% of the time.[28,29] Of course, this is not a method to be used for tumor bleeding from the proximal airway. It is appropriate for hemoptysis for bronchiectasis, lung cancer, arteriovenous malformations, and so forth. Complications from BAE are rare and minor. They include complications at femoral access sites (pseudoaneurysms, intimal dissection), small risk of stroke caused by embolization (this has become less common with superselective embolization), and the risk of rebleeding. The risk of rebleeding depends on the cause of the hemoptysis and the extent of embolization. Rebleeding is thought to occur because of the development of collaterals, distributaries that have not been embolized, or continuing inflammation. In cases of arteriovenous malformation, BAE represents definitive therapy in most cases. The extent of rebleeding is greater in bronchiectasis and aspergillomas and is higher still in lung cancer. Overall, 30-day rebleeding rates average at approximately 30% in large series. Therefore, definitive treatment should be planned for as soon as possible after embolization if patients are surgical candidates. Often, patients are not surgical candidates because of poor lung function or inoperable cancer. In the case of cancer, radiation therapy is a good palliative option. In inoperable cases with benign disease, repeat BAE can be performed to achieve reasonable long-term results.

A brief note of the treatment of aorto-bronchial fistulae deserves mention. Surgical repair of this difficult problem has prohibitive mortality. Endovascular stent-graft technology has revolutionized the treatment of this problem by decreasing the morbidity and mortality of treatment and is the treatment of choice if patients can be stabilized enough to be a candidate for such therapy.[30] Unfortunately, deployment of a stent graft in the setting of communication with infected bronchus may result in an infected stent graft; thus, definitive surgery may also be required.

Surgery

In the event of massive hemoptysis, surgery remains the last resort for bleeding control. However, surgery in this scenario has a very high mortality (25%).[2] This risk can be reduced if the bleeding can be temporized with methods outlined earlier. Time gained this way should be used to assess the extent of resection that can be safely performed and optimize the medical condition of patients. Such semielective surgery still carries a risk higher than completely elective cases but dramatically less than that performed in the emergency setting. Recent series have demonstrated that such semielective operations can be performed with mortality rates approaching routine elective resections.[31,32]

SUMMARY

Massive hemoptysis is a surgical problem that is not uncommon. A systematic yet flexible and multidisciplinary approach leads to optimal outcomes. The initial focus should be on stabilizing patients and securing the airway. This effort should be followed by methods to stop the bleeding, preferably nonsurgical methods. These methods should be followed by consideration for definitive therapy, including surgical therapy for appropriate patients.

REFERENCES

1. Corey R, Hla KM. Major and massive hemoptysis: reassessment of conservative management. Am J Med Sci 1987;294(5):301–9.
2. Garzon AA, Cerruti MM, Golding ME. Exsanguinating hemoptysis. J Thorac Cardiovasc Surg 1982; 84(6):829–33.

3. Sakr L, Dutau H. Massive hemoptysis: an update on the role of bronchoscopy in diagnosis and management. Respiration 2010;80(1):38–58.
4. Ibrahim WH. Massive haemoptysis: the definition should be revised. Eur Respir J 2008;32(4):1131–2.
5. Flume PA, Yankaskas JR, Ebeling M, et al. Massive hemoptysis in cystic fibrosis. Chest 2005;128(2):729–38.
6. Ong TH, Eng P. Massive hemoptysis requiring intensive care. Intensive Care Med 2003;29(2):317–20.
7. Valipour A, Kreuzer A, Koller H, et al. Bronchoscopy-guided topical hemostatic tamponade therapy for the management of life-threatening hemoptysis. Chest 2005;127(6):2113–8.
8. Conlan AA, Hurwitz SS. Management of massive haemoptysis with the rigid bronchoscope and cold saline lavage. Thorax 1980;35(12):901–4.
9. Binesh F, Samet M, Bovanlu TR. A case of pulmonary carcinoid tumour in a pregnant woman successfully treated with bronchoscopic (electrocautery) therapy. BMJ Case Rep 2013;2013 [pii:bcr2013009250].
10. Tsukamoto T, Sasaki H, Nakamura H. Treatment of hemoptysis patients by thrombin and fibrinogen-thrombin infusion therapy using a fiberoptic bronchoscope. Chest 1989;96(3):473–6.
11. Bense L. Intrabronchial selective coagulative treatment of hemoptysis. Report of three cases. Chest 1990;97(4):990–6.
12. Freitag L, Tekolf E, Stamatis G, et al. Three years experience with a new balloon catheter for the management of haemoptysis. Eur Respir J 1994;7(11):2033–7.
13. Jolliet P, Soccal P, Chevrolet JC. Control of massive hemoptysis by endobronchial tamponade with a pulmonary artery balloon catheter. Crit Care Med 1992;20(12):1730–2.
14. Kato R, Sawafuji M, Kawamura M, et al. Massive hemoptysis successfully treated by modified bronchoscopic balloon tamponade technique. Chest 1996;109(3):842–3.
15. Saw EC, Gottlieb LS, Yokoyama T, et al. Flexible fiberoptic bronchoscopy and endobronchial tamponade in the management of massive hemoptysis. Chest 1976;70(5):589–91.
16. Brandes JC, Schmidt E, Yung R. Occlusive endobronchial stent placement as a novel management approach to massive hemoptysis from lung cancer. J Thorac Oncol 2008;3(9):1071–2.
17. Coiffard B, Laroumagne S, Plojoux J, et al. Endobronchial occlusion for massive hemoptysis with a guidewire-assisted custom-made silicone spigot: a new technique. J Bronchology Interv Pulmonol 2014;21(4):366–8.
18. Dutau H, Palot A, Haas A, et al. Endobronchial embolization with a silicone spigot as a temporary treatment for massive hemoptysis: a new bronchoscopic approach of the disease. Respiration 2006;73(6):830–2.
19. Reisz G. Topical hemostatic tamponade: another tool in the treatment of massive hemoptysis. Chest 2005;127(6):1888–9.
20. Bhattacharyya P, Dutta A, Samanta AN, et al. New procedure: bronchoscopic endobronchial sealing; a new mode of managing hemoptysis. Chest 2002;121(6):2066–9.
21. Sutedja G, Postmus PE. Bronchoscopic treatment of lung tumors. Lung Cancer 1994;11(1–2):1–17.
22. Morice RC, Ece T, Ece F, et al. Endobronchial argon plasma coagulation for treatment of hemoptysis and neoplastic airway obstruction. Chest 2001;119(3):781–7.
23. Han CC, Prasetyo D, Wright GM. Endobronchial palliation using Nd:YAG laser is associated with improved survival when combined with multimodal adjuvant treatments. J Thorac Oncol 2007;2(1):59–64.
24. Hetzel MR, Smith SG. Endoscopic palliation of tracheobronchial malignancies. Thorax 1991;46(5):325–33.
25. Maiwand MO, Asimakopoulos G. Cryosurgery for lung cancer: clinical results and technical aspects. Technol Cancer Res Treat 2004;3(2):143–50.
26. Zhikai Z, Lizhi N, Liang Z, et al. Treatment of central type lung cancer by combined cryotherapy: experiences of 47 patients. Cryobiology 2013;67(2):225–9.
27. Khalil A, Parrot A, Nedelcu C, et al. Severe hemoptysis of pulmonary arterial origin: signs and role of multidetector row CT angiography. Chest 2008;133(1):212–9.
28. Chen J, Chen LA, Liang ZX, et al. Immediate and long-term results of bronchial artery embolization for hemoptysis due to benign versus malignant pulmonary diseases. Am J Med Sci 2014;348(3):204–9.
29. Fruchter O, Schneer S, Rusanov V, et al. Bronchial artery embolization for massive hemoptysis: long-term follow-up. Asian Cardiovasc Thorac Ann 2015;23(1):55–60.
30. Wheatley GH 3rd, Nunez A, Preventza O, et al. Have we gone too far? Endovascular stent-graft repair of aortobronchial fistulas. J Thorac Cardiovasc Surg 2007;133(5):1277–85.
31. Alexander GR. A retrospective review comparing the treatment outcomes of emergency lung resection for massive haemoptysis with and without preoperative bronchial artery embolization. Eur J Cardiothorac Surg 2014;45(2):251–5.
32. Zhang Y, Chen C, Jiang GN. Surgery of massive hemoptysis in pulmonary tuberculosis: immediate and long-term outcomes. J Thorac Cardiovasc Surg 2014;148(2):651–6.

Great Vessel Injury in Thoracic Surgery

Manuel Villa, MD, Inderpal S. Sarkaria, MD*

KEYWORDS

• Bleeding control • Minimally invasive thoracic surgery • Mediastinoscopy • Lung resection • Thymectomy • Esophagectomy

KEY POINTS

- Prevention is the optimal method of dealing with intraoperative bleeding complications in thoracic surgery.
- Thorough preoperative workup, including review of relevant imaging, with a particular focus on normal and variant vascular anatomy, is important in detecting risk factors for bleeding.
- Preparedness for complications ensures an effective and expedited response when intraoperative bleeding presents, especially in settings with limited access to the injury.
- Once bleeding occurs, continuous communication with the surgical team and immediate availability of surgical instruments and blood products are fundamental for an effective and successful response to the event.

INTRAOPERATIVE BLEEDING IN GENERAL THORACIC SURGERY

Due to the nature of vascular structures within the chest, including complex anatomy and high rates of blood flow often involving a significant portion of the cardiac output, injury can result in significant and life-threatening blood loss within seconds of occurring. Effective and expedited treatment is key to preventing poor outcomes in these events.

Vascular injuries during open surgery are addressed through the same incision with few exceptions, such as transhiatal esophagectomy and mediastinoscopy. During minimally invasive procedures, decision factors regarding the best incision to perform include adequate access to the vascular injury, as well as the ability to complete the index procedure. **Tables 1** and **2** summarize procedure-specific vascular injury risks and injury-specific incisions for exposure.[1]

During an intraoperative bleeding event, basic principles include obtaining proximal and distal vascular control, assessment of injury, and repair. In general, injuries less than 30% of the vessel circumference can be repaired primarily; injuries between 30% and 50% of the vessel circumference may be patch repaired with elements such as vein, pericardium, or prosthetic materials; and injuries involving more than 50% of the circumference require either end-to-end anastomosis (if length is adequate), conduit interposition, or ligation.

Preoperative Imaging and Vascular Anatomic Variation

Preoperative imaging, especially computed tomography (CT), provides a valuable opportunity to identify vascular anatomic variations and understand tumor location with respect to major

The authors have nothing to disclose.
Department of Cardiothoracic Surgery, University of Pittsburgh Medical Center, Pittsburgh, PA, USA
* Corresponding author. Department of Cardiothoracic Surgery, University of Pittsburgh Medical Center, UPMC Presbyterian-Shadyside, 5200 Centre Avenue, Suite 715.27, Pittsburgh, PA 15232.
E-mail address: sarkariais@upmc.edu

Thorac Surg Clin 25 (2015) 261–278
http://dx.doi.org/10.1016/j.thorsurg.2015.04.001
1547-4127/15/$ – see front matter

Table 1
Procedure-related potential causes of bleeding

Procedure	Vascular Structure in Risk
Mediastinoscopy	Innominate artery SVC Azygous vein Main pulmonary artery Hilar pulmonary artery Ascending aorta
Lung resection	Pulmonary vessels Bronchial arteries Descending thoracic aorta Subclavian artery
Transhiatal esophagectomy	Inferior pulmonary vein Aortoesophageal branches Short gastric vessels
Transthoracic esophagectomy	Aortoesophageal branches Bronchial arteries Azygous vein
Thymectomy	Innominate vein SVC Internal thoracic vessels

Abbreviation: SVC, superior vena cava.

vascular structures. It is estimated that 95% to 98% of the vascular anatomy pertinent to the surgical procedure can be accurately determined preoperatively by CT.[2–5] The presence of calcification affecting lymph nodes has been associated with increased risk of vascular injury and a cause of conversion. Samson and colleagues[6] reported that patients with evidence of calcifications involving the hilum had a 37% risk of conversion, and a 25% risk of conversion with calcifications involving the bronchial tree.

Variations in the pulmonary arterial branching pattern are common and often may be the cause of bleeding complications when unrecognized, such as a posterior ascending artery originating from the superior segmental artery, and the wide variation in number of arterial branches to the left upper lobe. Although less common, venous abnormalities also have been recognized as a potential cause of vascular complications. The most common is locating a pulmonary segmental vein takeoff posterior to the bronchus intermedius, which is critical to recognize during subcarinal lymph node dissection.[7]

This finding was detected in 41 patients (5.7%) in a review of 725 CTs, and in 9 patients (3.9%) of 230 thoracotomy cases, with 55% draining to the upper pulmonary vein, 41% to the inferior pulmonary vein, and 4% to the superior segmental vein.[8] The number and distribution of the pulmonary venous drainage is also variable. In a review of 201 CT scans, Marom and colleagues[9] identified 2 primary right-sided pulmonary veins in 71% of patients, with the middle lobe vein joining the superior vein in 68%, and the inferior vein in 3%. In 28% of the patients there were between 3 and 5 pulmonary veins identified, and a single

Table 2
Recommended incisions to approach specific vascular injuries

Vascular Structure	Incision	Useful Measures
Innominate artery	Median sternotomy	Division of the innominate vein may offer better exposure
Innominate vein	Median sternotomy	Ligation for complex injuries is well tolerated
Superior vena cava	Median sternotomy	Fluid loading and vasoactive agents as required if cross clamping the SVC to be performed
Ascending aorta and aortic arch	Median sternotomy	—
Descending aorta	Left posterolateral thoracotomy	Left heart bypass may be required for complex injuries
Azygous vein	Right thoracotomy	—
Pulmonary vessels	Posterolateral thoracotomy	Intrapericardial vascular control sometimes may be required
Subclavian artery		
Left	Left anterolateral thoracotomy	Left posterolateral thoracotomy to be considered, may allow both repairing the injury and performing the index operation
Right	Median sternotomy	—

Adapted from Wall MJ Jr, Tsai P, Mattox KL. Heart and thoracic vascular injuries. In: Mattox KL, Moore EE, Feliciano DV, editors. Trauma. 7th edition. New York: McGraw Hill; 2013. p. 502.

pulmonary venous trunk in 2%. On the left side, 86% of the patients had 2 pulmonary veins and a single vein was present in 14%. Akiba and colleagues[10] reported their findings on 140 patients undergoing video-assisted thoracoscopic surgery (VATS) with high-resolution preoperative CT angiography. On the right side, 10% of patients had 3 venous trunks, and 4% had 4 or 5 venous trunks. Independent drainage of the middle lobe was present in 8%, and there was a common venous trunk in 13% of the patients. On the left, a common ostium was found in 33% of the patients.

Less common venous drainage abnormalities reported include a common ostium for the left and right inferior pulmonary veins,[11,12] a lingular vein draining to the lower pulmonary vein,[13] a lateral segment vein of the middle lobe draining to the inferior pulmonary vein, and a superior segment vein draining directly into the left atrium.[4,14] Given the variability in the pulmonary venous drainage, some investigators have recommended routine formal preoperative venous system assessment with CT in all patients.[15]

Some investigators have reported on the utility of preoperative CT for surgical planning[16] before thymectomy. Preoperative identification of venous drainage to the subclavian and variants may be useful especially for minimally invasive thymectomy.

Redo sternotomy is traditionally associated with significant risk of injury to vital structures such as aorta, right atrium, innominate vein, cardiac vascular grafts, right ventricle, and pulmonary artery, with reported mortality as high as 26%. Preoperative planning with CT has been shown to decrease the incidence of reentry injury.[17,18]

Minimally Invasive Thoracic Surgery and Intraoperative Bleeding

Most misadventures during minimally invasive thoracic surgery are attributed to the 2-dimensional view with absence of depth perception. Surgeons generally adapt to these limitations with largely unconscious techniques, such as object interposition, relative motion, shadow perspective, and expectation with continuous assessment of characteristics like texture variation, texture gradients (distribution of the direction of edges), and known object sizes, among others. These elements, combined with surgical maneuvers such as alternating far and close views as well as obtaining different perspectives with the camera from different ports, provide valuable information that can closely approximate a 3-dimensional view.[19,20]

Current robotic-assisted surgical systems provide stereoscopic vision in which each eye is presented a separate image of the same object, thus providing the benefit of direct depth perception.[21] Conversely, the main disadvantage of robotic-assisted surgery may be the absence of haptic feedback, although training and adaptation through development of "visual tension" may largely overcome this.[22–28] Also, the optical advantage of robotic-assisted approaches must be weighed against the risk of separating the surgeon from the immediate operative field, which may delay the time to definitive therapy in bleeding emergencies in the absence of an able bedside assistant.

Technical details and recommendations regarding safe performance of minimally invasive thoracic surgery and addressing intraoperative complications have been published.[29–34] Measures that have been shown to be useful are the designation of a dedicated minimally invasive thoracic surgery team and the availability of appropriate instrumentation and equipment at the time of emergency.

Once significant intraoperative bleeding occurs, immediate control of hemorrhage, ideally with direct compression, or alternatively with vascular clamping, must be established along with adequate visualization. If this cannot be accomplished, immediate conversion via the most expeditious route should be considered to prevent imminent exsanguination. If controlled, an assessment of need for conversion to open versus minimally invasive repair of the injury should be made. Conversion should be considered the most "conservative" method, and a low threshold for conversion maintained unless the surgeon is skilled and comfortable with techniques of minimally invasive vascular repair, such as intracorporeal vessel isolation, suturing, and tying. Immediate bleeding control is generally obtained with gauze compression ("sponge on a stick") and is often adequate given the low pressures within the pulmonary arterial and venous systems. Packing the chest or abdomen through utility incisions may also be an expeditious temporizing measure, allowing time for definitive exposure and repair. Once bleeding is under control and decision made to convert, the surgical field should be kept continuously displayed on a monitor while the incision is made.

In a 9-year review at a single institution, it was noticed that with increasing experience, the conversion rate from VATS to open dropped from 28% to 11%. Of 1227 patients who underwent lobectomy, 517 (42%) were performed VATS, 87 (7%) were converted to open, and 623 (51%) were performed via thoracotomy; 25% of the conversions (22 patients) were due to vascular injuries,

15 were due to pulmonary artery injury, 6 were due to pulmonary vein injury, and 1 was due to azygous vein injury.[35]

Device Malfunction

Estimates of device failure are derived mainly from the Food and Drug Administration Manufacturer and User Facility Device Experience (MAUDE) voluntary reporting system. True device malfunctions are relatively rare, with most likely due to operator error. However, routine precautions against device failures involving critical vascular structures, and familiarity with device-specific failsafe mechanisms and protocols, are important in troubleshooting these rare occurrences.

The vast majority of malfunctions associated with bleeding complications involve vascular stapling devices. In a review of the MAUDE database between 1992 and 2001, 17,687 reports of device malfunction were filed, with 2180 patients reported injured and 112 deaths associated with stapler malfunction; 21 of the deaths (18.8%) were in patients undergoing thoracic surgical procedures. The following were the most common failures reported: staples did not form 32%, device failure or malfunction 22%, suture line separation 19%, staple did not fire properly 11%, and sticking 6%.[36]

A more recent report found a 0.003% incidence of malfunction, with partial stapler fire, misfire, and failure to release the most common malfunctions identified. Results from one survey indicate that 86% of minimally invasive surgeons have experienced an incident in which the linear stapler would not release (66%) or not fire (73%) after application, with 25% having to significantly alter the planned operative procedure because of the malfunction.[37] Yano and colleagues[38] reported a single institution experience of 9 adverse events out of 3393 stapler deployments (**Fig. 1**). Eight were intraoperative and including significant oozing from the staple line, stapler failure, laceration of vasculature during stapler compression, and technical injury during stapler insertion. Cases of stapler sharp division without deployment of staples also have been reported.[39,40]

More recently, reports using the MAUDE database have focused on robotic system instrument failures, although it is unclear what proportion of these involved bleeding emergencies. A review focusing on patient injury and device failure found an estimated failure rate of 0.38%, with 4.8% of 189 device malfunctions associated with patient injury and no associated mortality.[41] Lucas and colleagues[42] reported an incidence of injuries related to robot malfunction of 2.3% for the period 2003 to 2006 and 3.1% for the period 2007 to 2009 with 1.6% and 0.2% mortality, respectively. In a review of the MAUDE database from 2009 to 2010 investigating unrecoverable faults of the robotic system, there were 528 reports of 565 failures; 285 were due to wrist or tool tip failures,

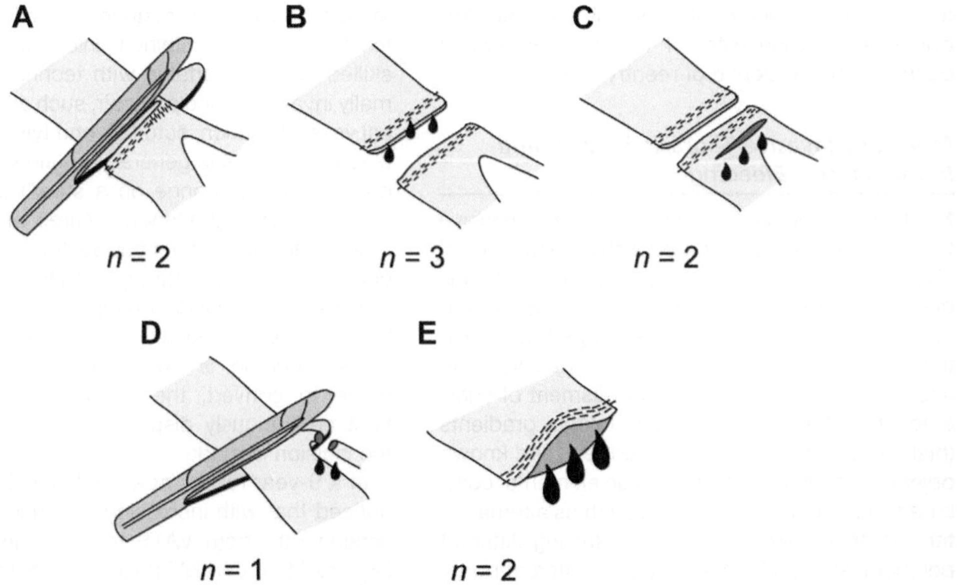

Fig. 1. Adverse events during pulmonary vascular stapling: (*A*) stapling failure, (*B*) persistent oozing, (*C*) laceration of adjacent vessels, (*D*) vascular injury during stapler insertion, and (*E*) dehiscence of staple line. (*From* Yano M, Takao M, Fujinaga T, et al. Adverse events of pulmonary vascular stapling in thoracic surgery. Interact Cardiovasc Thorac Surg 2013;17(2):281; with permission.)

174 due to cautery instrument failures with 90% involving arcing incidents, and 76 were instrument shaft failures such as material breaking off the shaft, splintering, or cracking.[43] However, the association of these failures as causative factors of hemorrhage is unknown and likely small.

PROCEDURE-SPECIFIC BLEEDING

Lung Resection

Overview

Preoperative identification and awareness of case-specific and patient-specific risk factors may help prevent hemorrhagic complications in most lung resections. These factors include body habitus, preoperative chemotherapy and radiation, previous surgery, lymph node calcification and/or granulomatous disease, tumor size, location, and relation to vascular structures, and metastatic lymph node involvement. It is important to either confirm the presence of normal anatomy or to identify relevant vascular anatomic variants or anomalies. These often may be recognized on preoperative imaging, in which modern radiographic reconstruction techniques may be of particular help.

Proper handling, loading, and cleansing of the surgical staplers in conjunction with refined stapling techniques also may preempt many injuries. These techniques include adequate vascular dissection and exposure, optimal stapler alignment, and stable and controlled stapler deployment without excessive tissue traction or tension during ligation, division, and withdrawal. The operating room team should be informed about critical parts of the dissection. Gauze or sponge on a stick should be on the table for immediate use, blood products available, and equipment and instruments for open surgery within reach during minimally invasive operations. Once bleeding occurs, the general principles of treatment are bleeding control, assessment of injury, and repair.

Overall, open and minimally invasive lung resections have been associated with low operative mortality and low incidence of intraoperative bleeding. The incidence of major bleeding in open lung resection has been reported at approximately 5%.[44] A more recent review of a national database with more than 33,095 patients who underwent lobectomy between 2008 and 2010 found an incidence of intraoperative bleeding of 1.9% for open, 1.3% for VATS, and 1.7% for robotic-assisted resections.[45] A large published series with 1100 VATS anatomic resections reported 7 conversions due to intraoperative bleeding and no intraoperative deaths.[46] In a review of literature on safety and efficacy, robotic-assisted lobectomy was comparable to VATS, with robotic conversion to open in a range of 1.0% to 19.2% (mean 8.7%).[47,48]

Cerfolio and colleagues[49] reported their experience on 106 robotic resections with 2 conversions for bleeding: one for pulmonary arterial bleeding to the anterior apical truncus during right upper lobectomy controlled with packing while converting, and another with parenchymal bleeding resulting from stapling during right upper lobe posterior segmentectomy. Park and colleagues[31] reported on 3 patients converted for minor bleeding events in a series of 325 robotic lobectomies, all initially controlled with direct "sponge-stick" compression through a utility incision while thoracotomy was performed.

Flores and colleagues,[50] in a series of 633 VATS lobectomies from Memorial Sloan-Kettering Cancer Center, reported on 12 cases experiencing "catastrophic" complications. In 2 patients with pulmonary arterial injury, pneumonectomy was ultimately required for salvage. Two patients underwent primary pulmonary anastomosis after inadvertent stapler transection of the right main pulmonary artery during right upper lobectomy. Similarly, another patient required reanastomosis of the left inferior pulmonary vein after stapling of a common trunk to both the inferior and superior veins. An intraoperative staple line dehiscence on the inferior pulmonary vein with retraction of the vessel into the pericardium required emergent thoracotomy for bleeding control, and in another to control bleeding to an azygo-caval junction injury caused during dissection of right paratracheal lymph nodes. One patient experienced subdiaphragmatic injury to the spleen manifesting as postoperative hypotension and requiring splenectomy. Similarly, Augustin and colleagues[51] reported on a patient experiencing subdiaphragmatic liver injury while undergoing minimally invasive mediastinal lymph node dissection.

Less common clinical scenarios

Cardiac tamponade, although rare, has been associated with bleeding complications after lung resection. Tovar[52] reported a case of tamponade that occurred during left lower lobectomy for a central tumor after clamping of the inferior pulmonary vein close to the pericardium. Sudden hemodynamic collapse ensued with injury and free bleeding of the vein that had retracted into the pericardium requiring intrapericardial control and repair. McLean and colleagues[53] reported on a patient with hemodynamic collapse secondary to tamponade 5 hours after right upper lobectomy due to a bleeding aberrant bronchial artery that had retracted into the pericardium. Ozawa and colleagues[54] reported a case of cardiac tamponade caused by injury of a branch of the circumflex artery during left anatomic segmental resection. Chen and colleagues[55] reported a direct injury to the left ventricle caused by a staple line.

Surgical technique

Particular attention to the vascular dissection and a refined stapling technique are of the highest importance to prevent bleeding complications. Avoiding application of clips that could interfere with proper stapler firing, ensuring proper stapler alignment, ensuring additional dissection around vessels to maximize unrestricted stapler passage, and avoiding tension or traction during device deployment are key components in preventing injury, which often occurs at branching points.[30,32] Vascular injury during introduction of the stapler is one of the most frequent mechanisms of injury. Dunning and Walker[56] reported a left main pulmonary artery injury during introduction of the stapler, in which "swab-on-a-stick" was used to control bleeding followed by thoracotomy and repair with pericardial patch.

Suggested techniques to increase the safety of stapler passage include use of a red-rubber catheter (8–14 French) or a Penrose drain to guide the anvil, or use of silk sutures or vessel loops to maximize the space for anvil passage around the vessels.[29,57,58]

Due to the low pressure pulmonary system, control of minor bleeding or oozing from staple lines, minor vasculature injuries, or parenchymal injuries often may be addressed adequately with a period of applied pressure. Different methods of pressure application have been described including use of a sponge or swab on a clamp or "stick" (most common),[46,56] suction-compression,[34] and closing the stapler on the bleeding source.[29,40,59] Use of electrocautery, clips, and other hemostatic agents also may be useful. Proximal vascular control is most often obtained around the main pulmonary arteries and can be accomplished intrapericardially if needed for proximal or complex injuries. Distal control occasionally can be obtained directly on the artery or vein of interest, but generally is performed at the level of the pulmonary veins, and also can be performed intrapericardially if needed.[60]

Minimally invasive vascular control of the pulmonary artery has been described and recommended by some investigators either as a preemptive maneuver when difficult dissection is expected, or for vascular control if bleeding presents. Vascular control can be obtained using silk sutures, vessel loops, or vascular clamps (**Figs. 2–4**).[61–64] Once bleeding is under control, assessment of the injury will determine the type of repair. The need for conversion should be considered early in minimally invasive operations. Experience from trauma and complex bronchovascular reconstruction techniques are helpful in weighing options for repair of inadvertent vascular injuries. Common options for vascular injury repair are primary closure, use of

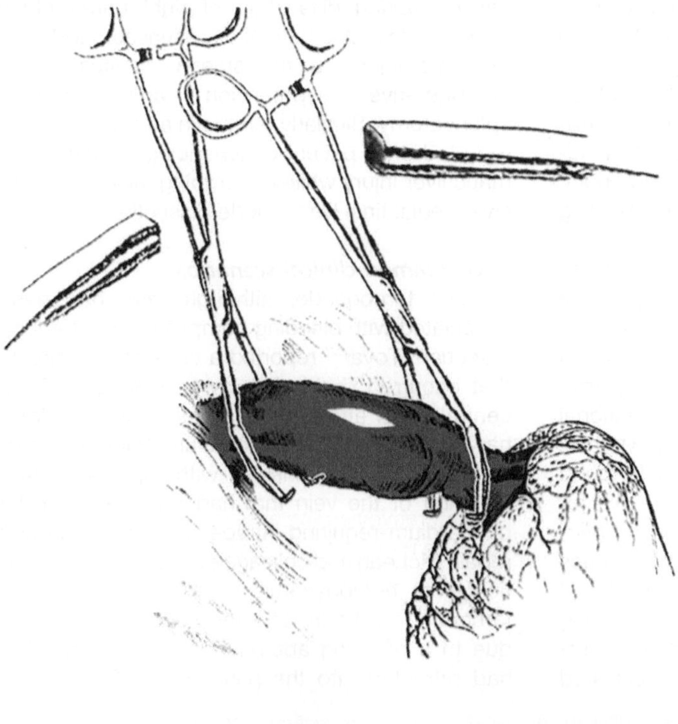

Fig. 2. Direct proximal and distal vascular control of pulmonary artery during VATS. (*From* Nakanishi R, Yamashita T, Oka S. Initial experience of video-assisted thoracic surgery lobectomy with partial removal of the pulmonary artery. Interact Cardiovasc Thorac Surg 2008;7:997; with permission. Published by European Association for Cardio-Thoracic Surgery. All rights reserved.)

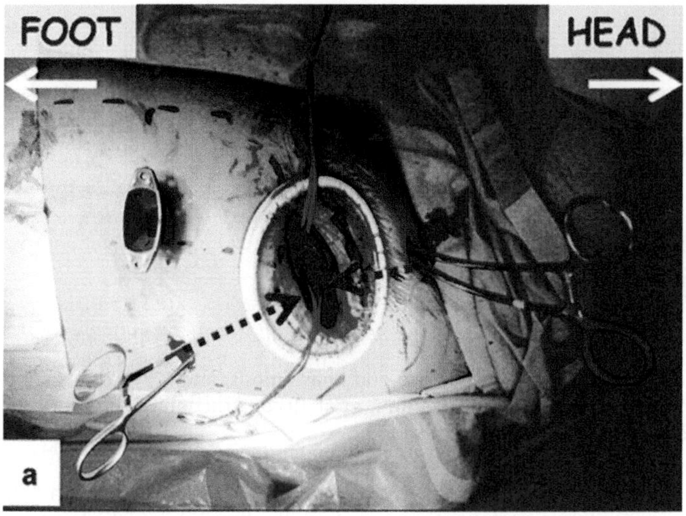

Fig. 3. Pulmonary artery control during VATS. The exterior appearance of our technique using DeBakey vascular clamps with double angle jaws through two 1-cm access incisions viewed from directly above (a) and edge-on. The pathway of the vascular clamps (*blue dotted lines*) involves "outside-field clamping," which avoids obstructing the limited visual field through the working port. (*Adapted from* Kamiyoshihara M, Nagashima T, Ibe T, et al. A tip for controlling the main pulmonary artery during video-assisted thoracic major pulmonary resection: the outside-field vascular clamping technique. Interact Cardiovasc Thorac Surg 2010;11(5):694; with permission. Published by European Association for Cardio-Thoracic Surgery. All rights reserved.)

patch, end-to-end anastomosis, and use of conduit (**Fig. 5**). Primary repair is reserved for injuries smaller than one-third of the circumference of the vessel. Vascular patches are tailored to the defect with commonly described materials being autologous pericardium, bovine pericardium, and azygous vein. Common conduit options include autologous pericardium, pulmonary vein, or polytetra-fluoro-ethylene (PTFE). Attention must be paid to the length of the conduit to prevent kinking or rotation after lung reexpansion. In the presence of concomitant airway injuries, use of interposition muscle flaps is useful to prevent broncho-arterial fistulas.[65–69]

Complex repair of the pulmonary vein is occasionally required and frequently associated with stapling of a common trunk of the left pulmonary vein. Primary end-to-end anastomosis,[50] use of a vein cuff from the pulmonary vein of the resected lobe,[70] and use of pericardial patch[71] have been reported.

Most complex repairs are performed by thoracotomy, but recent reports have described minimally invasive approaches to repair of these injuries.[72,73]

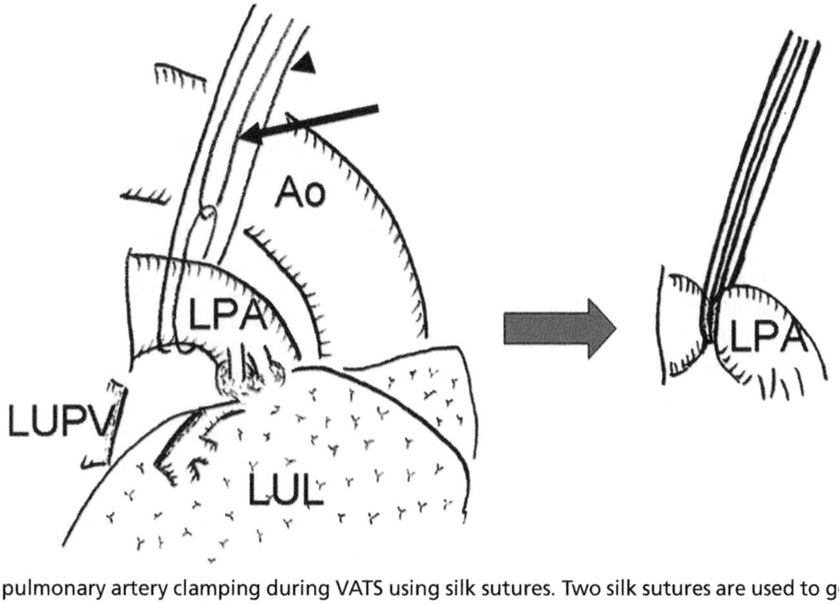

Fig. 4. Main pulmonary artery clamping during VATS using silk sutures. Two silk sutures are used to get control of the pulmonary artery (*Arrow* and *arrowhead*). Ao, aorta; LPA, left pulmonary artery; LUL, left upper lobe; LUPV, left upper pulmonary vein. (*From* Watanabe A, Koyanagi T, Nakashima S, et al. How to clamp the main pulmonary artery during video-assisted thoracoscopic surgery lobectomy. Eur J Cardiothorac Surg 2007;31(1):130; with permission.)

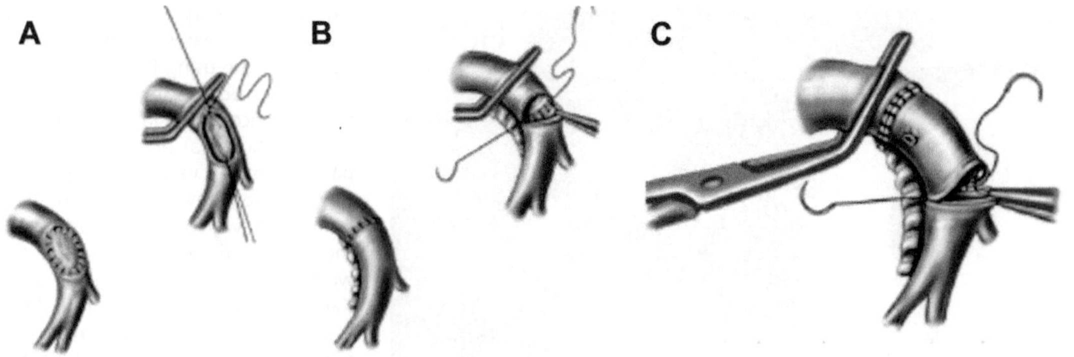

Fig. 5. Pulmonary artery repair: (*A*) pericardial patch repair, (*B*) end-to-end anastomosis, and (*C*) reconstruction with autologous conduit. (*Adapted from* Ibrahim M, Maurizi G, Venuta F, et al. Reconstruction of the bronchus and pulmonary artery. Thorac Surg Clin 2013;23:337–47; with permission.)

Consequences

The short-term and long-term outcomes of minimally invasive lung resection seem not to be affected by conversion to open surgery. Jones and colleagues[74] reported on 286 patients on whom VATS was attempted for cancer, of which 30 patients were converted to open (10.4%) and 4 patients with metastatic disease were excluded. There was no difference in short-term or long-term surgical outcomes. Eleven conversions were for bleeding (37%) and 2 for stapler misfire (7%); types of injury and treatment were not specified for the remaining cases.

Two other reports found differences in operating time, blood loss, and length of stay, but no differences in complication, survival, and recurrence rates.[75,76]

Extrapleural Pneumonectomy for Mesothelioma

Because of the significant pleural thickening associated with malignant pleural mesothelioma, extrapleural dissection carries the potential for significant intrathoracic vascular injury. Almost every vascular structure is at risk if caution is not practiced with constant reassessment of anatomy and spatial relationships throughout the course of dissection. In the left chest, the internal mammary vessels, subclavian artery, and aorta are at risk. In the right chest, particular attention must be paid during the diaphragmatic dissection, when phrenic veins are at risk and excessive traction can tear the inferior vena cava. The azygous vein and superior vena cava also are at risk.[77,78]

Decortication

As previously mentioned, decortication in particular situations of thickened pleura and fibrothorax carries the risk of potential vascular injuries. Rai and colleagues[79] reported a left subclavian artery injury during a decortication in a patient with a chronic pleural empyema.

Mediastinal Procedures

Thymectomy

Overall, bleeding complications during mediastinal resections are rare. Masaoka and colleagues[80] reported a 20-year experience of 384 thymectomies with no operative deaths and no major intraoperative bleeding complications.[80,81] Similar outcomes were reported by Shrager and colleagues[82,83] using extended transcervical approach on 164 patients with no intraoperative bleeding complications. Roviaro and colleagues[84] reported their experience from 1991 to 1999 on 71 VATS for mediastinal pathology with 1 intraoperative bleeding event controlled thoracoscopically (not specified how) and 2 early postoperative bleeding events, one requiring open control of a port-site intercostal arterial injury. No active bleeding was found on exploration in the second patient.

The most common cause of bleeding during minimally invasive thymectomy is injury to the thymic veins or the innominate vein, although others do occur. Cerfolio and Bryant[33] reported conversion for bleeding during robotic resection of a 10-cm middle mediastinal tumor secondary to a superior vena cava injury controlled with packing, followed by primary repair requiring open conversion. In a series of 33 patients undergoing robotic-assisted mediastinal resections, including 22 thymectomies, Augustin and colleagues[51] described 2 conversions for bleeding, including a subdiaphragmatic liver injury, and bleeding from the internal mammary artery. Whitson and colleagues[85] described technical details for a safe thoracoscopic thymectomy, including optimal patient positioning, availability of separate video camera and thoracoscope set up for left phrenic visualization, dissection with electrocautery and harmonic scalpels, use of low-level of CO2 insufflation to improve exposure and dissection of areolar tissues, and circumferential dissection and ligation of thymic veins. Division of the thymic veins with energy sources such as the harmonic scalpel have been described without bleeding complications, although most surgeons prefer application of hemostatic clips before division of the veins for assured mechanical occlusion of the vessels.[86]

Mediastinoscopy

Overall, mediastinoscopy has a low incidence of bleeding of 0% to 0.6% and low mortality 0% to 0.2%.[87–90] In a series of 3391 mediastinoscopies over 12 years, Park and colleagues[90] reported 14 major bleeding complications. Initial management in all cases was packing of the mediastinal tunnel followed by sternotomy in 9 and right posterolateral thoracotomy in 5. There was 1 postoperative death. The injured structures were related to initial dissection and exposure, and to the nodal stations being sampled. Sternotomy was performed in 5 patients with innominate artery injury incurred during initial dissection. Azygous vein injury was sustained in 3 patients and superior vena cava injury in 1 patient during right paratracheal (station 4R) biopsy. Two were approached with posterolateral thoracotomy and one by median sternotomy. The caval injury was approached by combined partial sternotomy and anterolateral thoracotomy (hemi-clamshell incision). Subcarinal (station 7) dissection–related injuries included 2 to the right main pulmonary artery approached with median sternotomy and anterolateral thoracotomy, and 1 bronchial artery injury approached through posterolateral thoracotomy. There were 2 injuries during dissection of the right hilar lymph nodes (station 10R) to arterial branches to the right upper lobe.

Mediastinoscopy and the complex mediastinum The complex mediastinum has been variably defined as those having undergone previous mediastinoscopy or other mediastinal procedures, radiation or chemotherapy, or previous sternotomy.

Previous mediastinoscopy, radiation, or chemotherapy may increase the difficulty of the dissection and has been associated with increased morbidity and mortality. Although mortality and morbidity for first time mediastinoscopy has been reported at 0.05% and 1%,[91,92] these rates have been reported as high as 1% and 3% to 8% in the complex mediastinum.[93–95] Louie and colleagues[96] reported on 75 mediastinoscopies performed on patients with complex mediastinum including 15 redo mediastinoscopies, 45 after combined chemoradiation, 6 after radiotherapy alone, and 9 after chemotherapy alone. Although overall considered feasible, they reported 1 vascular injury to the azygous vein approached through a right thoracotomy, and 2 mediastinoscopies aborted because of severe fibrosis. De Waele and colleagues[93] reported 104 redo mediastinoscopies, of which 79 patients had received chemotherapy and 25 chemoradiation. Mortality was 1% and morbidity 2%. There was 1 intraoperative death from bleeding at the origin of the innominate artery (brachiocephalic trunk), complicated with hemopericardium and cardiac arrest; 1 bleeding from bronchial artery that was controlled with packing; and 1 injury to the superior vena cava (SVC) required right thoracotomy and primary repair.

Although a previous sternotomy may not preclude mediastinoscopy, the surgeon should be prepared for the need for redo sternotomy in the event of major bleeding. Access to cardiopulmonary bypass and peripheral cannulation techniques are often advised in the approach of these patients should conversion to an open approach be necessary.

Surgical technique and specific injuries Avoiding the application of excessive traction while manipulating the mediastinoscope and during biopsy, and using needle aspiration to confirm the nonvascular nature of unclear biopsy targets are recommended to prevent injuries. If bleeding ensues, packing with gauze and pressure applied either with mediastinoscope or digital compression is the best initial step,[89] and may be adequate to definitively control hemorrhage. If inadequate control is achieved, then an alternative surgical approach should be expeditiously pursued based on the exposure required to repair the injury and, if feasible, complete the index operation.[90]

Superior vena cava injury Optimal exposure is obtained with median sternotomy or combined partial sternotomy and right anterolateral thoracotomy (hemi-clamshell). Most injuries are small, encompassing less than 30% of the circumference of the vessel. Primary repair with lateral venorrhaphy is often sufficient. Complex injuries may require patch repair or conduit interposition. Autologous patches are commonly used: pericardium, azygous, saphenous, or pulmonary veins have been described. Reconstruction techniques used during elective vascular oncologic resections may be valuable to consider in more complex repairs (**Fig. 6**). Described conduit choices include cryopreserved arterial allografts,[97] PTFE,[98–101]

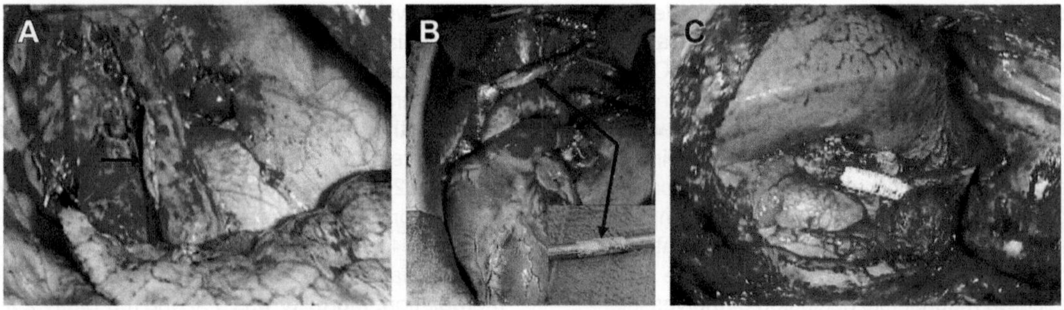

Fig. 6. Superior vena cava repair: (*A*) patch repair, the *arrow* points to the pericardial patch used for repair. (*B*) reconstruction with custom-made autologous pericardium conduit, the *lower arrow* points to the custom-made pericardial tube. The *upper arrow* points to the pericardial tube in place after repair. (*C*) reconstruction with PTFE conduit. (*Adapted from* Spaggiari L, Leo F, Veronesi G, et al. Superior vena cava resection for lung and mediastinal malignancies: a single-center experience with 70 cases. Ann Thorac Surg 2007;83:223–30; with permission.)

and custom-made bovine pericardial tube.[99] Graft thrombosis is of particular concern, with reported thrombosis rates between 20% and 50%[98,102] for synthetics, and approximately 10%[99] for biologicals.

Innominate artery injury This devastating traction injury has been most associated with extended cervical mediastinoscopy with passage of the scope anterior to the aortic arch between the innominate and left carotid arteries.[90,103] Packing followed by immediate sternotomy is likely necessary to control bleeding and repair, which may require complex reconstruction depending on the extent of injury. The bypass technique as described by Johnston and colleagues[104] may be useful in dealing with this injury, given the injury is often incurred at its origin off the aorta (**Fig. 7**). Smith and colleagues[105] also described successful endovascular repair using aortic grafts for

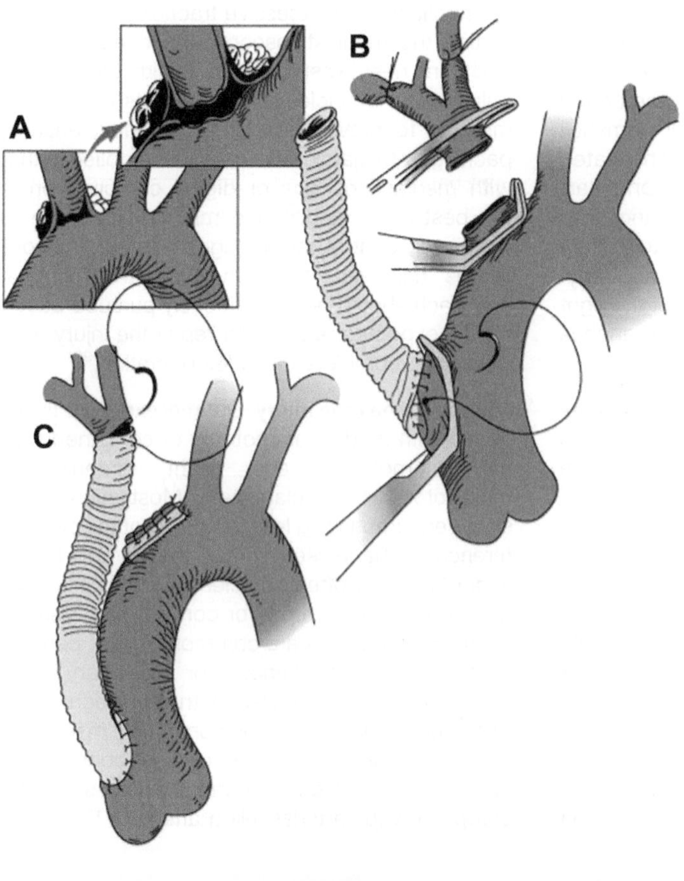

Fig. 7. The bypass technique for repair of innominate artery injuries. (*A*) Injury to the pericardial innominate artery. (*B*) Innominate artery is divided. (*C*) Bypass from proximal ascending aorta to the innominate artery. (*From* Johnston RH Jr, Wall MJ Jr, Mattox KL. Innominate artery trauma: a thirty-year experience. J Vasc Surg 1993;17(1):504; with permission.)

injuries to the origin of the brachiocephalic artery incurred during extended mediastinoscopy.

Azygous vein injury Most commonly injured during right pulmonary resection, esophagectomy, or mediastinoscopy, exposure is readily achieved through right thoracotomy. If primary repair is not feasible, ligation should be performed and is well tolerated (**Fig. 8**).[106]

Aortic injury Direct aortic injury during mediastinoscopy is rare, but has been described. Smith and colleagues[105] reported on a patient undergoing effective endovascular repair of an aortic injury after mediastinoscopy. The patient presented with a delayed aortic pseudoaneurysm after biopsy of the left paratracheal space. At the time of operation, intraoperative hemorrhage was controlled with packing and vascular clips and the patient completed palliative radiotherapy before repair.

Esophageal surgery

The risk of vascular injury during hiatal dissection has been well documented. Baigrie and colleagues[107] reported 3 injuries during dissection of the esophageal hiatus: aorta, large inferior phrenic vein, and inferior vena cava. Leggett and colleagues,[108] Yano and colleagues,[109] and Bonavina and colleagues[110] also reported on aortic injuries during esophageal procedures, including antireflux operations and esophagectomy. Injury to the left hepatic vein has been documented as well.[111]

Most reports of major thoracic bleeding complications during esophagectomy are associated with blunt dissection during transhiatal approaches. Although the reported incidence of major bleeding during transhiatal esophagectomy is less than 1%, the associated mortality with vascular injury can be as high as 40%. This risk may be increased in the presence of bulky, midthoracic tumors, and with preoperative radiotherapy. In a series of 2029 transhiatal esophagectomies, Orringer and colleagues[112] reported less than 1% incidence of intrathoracic hemorrhage, with 9 conversions to thoracotomy to control hemorrhage. Four patients with mediastinal bleeding died during surgery, attesting to the severity of these injuries.

Structures at risk during blunt mediastinal dissection include the inferior pulmonary veins, azygos vein, and aorta. Maintaining dissection toward these structures to minimize traction is advised. If bleeding occurs, initial maneuvers include mediastinal packing and compression through the hiatus if tolerated, visualization and assessment of ability to repair the injury through the hiatus, and Trendelenburg positioning. If thoracotomy is required, laterality may depend on the nature of the injury (for example, right vs left pulmonary veins) and the level of the esophagus being dissected. A left thoracotomy may provide better exposure to the lower third of the esophagus and aorta, and a right thoracotomy for the middle and upper esophagus, as well as the azygous vein.

In a review of 710 patients undergoing transhiatal resection, Javed and colleagues[113] reported an incidence of major bleeding of 1.4%. The associated mortality was 40%, with 2 intraoperative deaths. Univariate analysis identified midthoracic esophageal tumors and preoperative radiotherapy as risk factors for bleeding. The injuries reported were 4 to the descending thoracic aorta, 2 to aortoesophageal arteries, 3 to the azygous vein, and 1

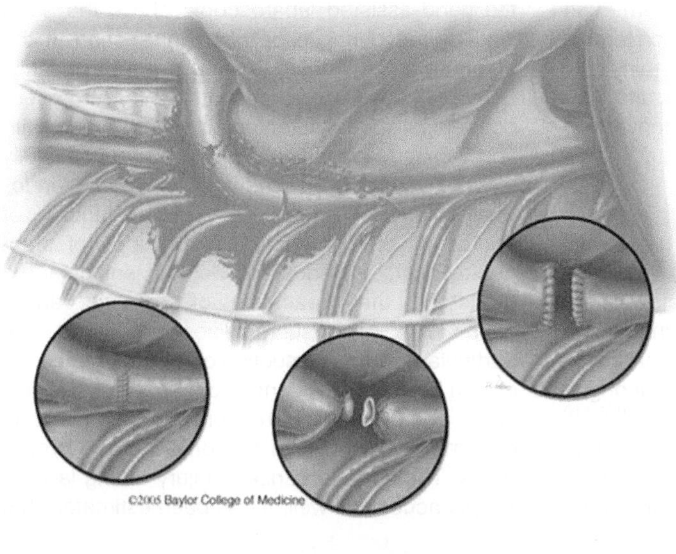

Fig. 8. Repair options for azygous vein injuries: primary repair, ligation or division, and oversewing. (*From* Wall MJ, Mattox KL, DeBakey ME. Injuries to the azygous venous system. J Trauma 2006;60:508; with permission.)

to the inferior pulmonary vein. Injuries were approached through right thoracotomy in 6 patients, left thoracotomy in 1, and bilateral thoracotomy in 1. Transhiatal repair was performed in 2 patients.

Transthoracic approaches to esophagectomy may allow the advantage of direct visualization of major vasculature in the chest, minimizing the need for blind dissection. These approaches also allow ready access for control and repair when necessary. The primary vascular structures at risk are identical to transhiatal approaches and include the azygous vein, inferior pulmonary vein, aortoesophageal branches, bronchial arteries, and aorta. Methods of specific repair are similar for those already described in this article.

Particular attention should be given to division of the short gastric vessels, which are the most common cause of intraoperative or early postoperative abdominal bleeding in these patients. It is during this portion of the gastric mobilization that the risk of splenic injury is highest, often caused by traction injury or direct injury to the splenic hilum due to poor visualization, particularly in obese patients.

Although rare, aberrant vasculature may increase the risk of bleeding. Pantvaidya and colleagues[114] reported a patient in whom an aberrant subclavian artery was transected during minimally invasive transthoracic esophagectomy. Repair was performed with PTFE interposition graft through median sternotomy.

Minimally invasive approaches to esophagectomy may improve visualization and decrease the risk of major bleeding events in experienced centers. In a recent review of the literature of 24 articles for a total of 257 patients who underwent minimally invasive robotic surgery of the mediastinum,[115] there was only one reported intraoperative bleeding complication from an aortoesophageal artery that required conversion to open surgery,[116] In a series of 1011 minimally invasive esophagectomies by Luketich and colleagues,[117] 6 patients (0.6%) required conversion for major bleeding complications.

Specific injuries

Aortic injury Aortic injury is most commonly described in association with esophageal procedures and resections, as well as parietal pleural decortication for cancer or complex infections. Although usually due to vessel trauma to bronchial or esophageal perforating arteries near their origin, direct aortic injury is also a concern.[77,78,107–110] Direct suture repair is often an option during open transthoracic resections, but also may require advanced aortic repair with patch repair, replacement, or reconstruction techniques with or without the need for cardiopulmonary bypass or deep hypothermia.

Given the anatomic location of the esophagus in close proximity to the aorta, esophageal surgery is associated with potential bleeding injuries of the aorta throughout all its length: neck, chest, and abdomen. Not only is the aorta at risk during the index procedure, but also in the postoperative period in the setting of anastomotic complications. Aortic erosion and bleeding have been reported in the setting of anastomotic leaks and associated infection, as well as after placement of endoluminal stents for treatment of these complications. Development of aortoesophageal or aortogastric fistulae is a feared and well-known complication involving a high operative mortality.[118–122] Endovascular stent graft repair of aortic complications due to esophagectomy have been reported, both in the immediate operative setting and in the postoperative period, often involving infected mediastinal fields with anastomotic leaks or fistulizing complications.[123–126] Matono and colleagues[127] reported a mortality in a patient undergoing open Ivor Lewis esophagectomy with development of a mediastinal abscess presenting with active bleeding through mediastinal drain. Chest CT identified a ruptured descending thoracic aorta pseudoaneurysm treated with endovascular repair and further complicated by aortobronchial fistula formation. The aortic stent graft could be seen with the bronchoscope. A case of ruptured pseudoaneurysm of the descending thoracic aorta was reported in a patient who had undergone esophagectomy through a left thoracotomy approach complicated by anastomotic leak and empyema. Endovascular aortic graft placement was successfully performed. In another patient who underwent Ivor Lewis esophagectomy, during the hand-assisted laparoscopic phase the aorta was injured during esophageal dissection at the diaphragmatic hiatus and was repaired primarily. On follow-up CT 6 months later, a 25-mm pseudoaneurysm was detected at the site of repair, and an endovascular stent was successfully placed. Caution is advised when embracing endovascular repair given the circumstances of contamination or infection in the area of stent deployment, analogous to deployment of aortic grafts in the treatment of mycotic aneurysms.[128,129] The supraceliac aorta is at risk particularly during dissection of the esophageal hiatus in both antireflux and esophageal cancer surgery, the thoracic surgeon should exercise extreme caution during this phase of the procedures. The aorta is at risk of injury during laparoscopic access as well. It has been estimated that

6.4% of the iatrogenic injuries during laparoscopic access involve the abdominal aorta.[107,130]

Supraceliac aortic vascular control The gastrohepatic omentum is incised, the stomach is retracted to the left and the aorta is identified and controlled either with a vascular clamp or using a mechanical aortic compressor. Incision of the right crus may be necessary for adequate exposure and clamp placement.[131] More complex injuries may require left medial visceral rotation. Initially described by DeBakey for thoracoabdominal aneurysm repair, this technique also has been used for emergent exposure in trauma and for repair of juxtarenal aortic aneurysms. Aortic exposure is achieved after transecting the avascular line of Toldt along the left colic gutter followed by en bloc medial rotation of the left colon, spleen, pancreas, and stomach.[132–134] Endovascular control with aortic occlusion balloons is another technique that also may be considered if direct control through the operative field cannot be accomplished.

Celiac trunk and branches The celiac trunk and its branches are at risk of injury during celiac dissection, lymphadenectomy, and left gastric vascular pedicle division. At this level, splenic artery injury can be treated with ligation without need for splenectomy given collateral flow from the superior mesenteric artery. More distal injuries to the splenic artery are best addressed by splenectomy. Direct celiac trunk injury will likely require primary repair or revascularization with conduit (indicated more commonly with hepatic artery injury). Although ligation of the celiac trunk has been well tolerated in young patients without significant atherosclerotic disease, bypass of the hepatic artery should be considered given the significant risk of severe liver ischemic complications. Injuries to the celiac trunk and its branches also may manifest postoperatively. Yau and colleagues[135] reported a case of celiac and mesenteric artery thrombosis in the postoperative period after laparoscopic antireflux surgery.

Spleen Splenic injury is often the result of excessive capsular traction during lysis of gastrosplenic attachments and associated left upper quadrant crural and diaphragmatic adhesions, and during mobilization of the gastric fundus with dissection and division of short gastric arteries. With a reported incidence of 4% to 9% during esophagectomy, splenectomy has been associated with increased rate of anastomotic leak, length of stay, and in-hospital mortality but with no significant effect on overall survival.[107,136–140] Numerous techniques for splenic repair have been reported including use of topical hemostatic agents, compressing the spleen with absorbable mesh, and pledgeted suture repair. Partial splenectomy may be feasible with injures restricted to one splenic segment or pole, but a low threshold for complete splenectomy should be maintained as a definitive maneuver. The risk for overwhelming postsplenectomy sepsis always should be considered and appropriate vaccination is recommended against *Streptococcus pneumoniae*, *Haemophilus influenzae*, and *Neisseria meningitides*.[141]

SUMMARY

Major intraoperative bleeding complications during general thoracic surgical procedures are relatively rare, and often can be avoided with careful preoperative planning, review of relevant imaging, and meticulous surgical technique. When they do occur, a prepared and methodical response with initial control of bleeding, assessment of injury, and appropriate repair are necessary to maximize outcomes. During minimally invasive operations requiring conversion to open surgery, the surgeon should be well versed in injury-specific incisions and approaches to maximize adequate exposure to the injury, and when feasible, allow completion of the index operation.

REFERENCES

1. Wall MJ Jr, Tsai P, Mattox KL. Chapter 26: heart and thoracic vascular injuries. In: Mattox KL, Moore EE, Feliciano DV, editors. Trauma. 7th edition. New York: McGraw Hill; 2013. p. 485–511.
2. Watanabe S, Arai K, Watanabe T, et al. Use of three-dimensional computed tomographic angiography of pulmonary vessels for lung resections. Ann Thorac Surg 2003;75:388–92.
3. Fukuhara K, Akashi A, Nakane S, et al. Preoperative assessment of the pulmonary artery by three-dimensional computed tomography before video-assisted thoracic surgery lobectomy. Eur J Cardiothorac Surg 2008;34:875–7.
4. Akiba T, Marushima H, Harada J, et al. Anomalous pulmonary vein detected using three-dimensional computed tomography in a patient with lung cancer undergoing thoracoscopic lobectomy. Gen Thorac Cardiovasc Surg 2008;56:413–6.
5. Akiba T, Marushima H, Harada J, et al. Importance of preoperative imaging with 64-row three-dimensional multidetector computed tomography for safer video-assisted thoracic surgery in lung cancer. Surg Today 2009;39:844–7.
6. Samson P, Guitron J, Reed MF, et al. Predictors of conversion to thoracotomy for video-assisted thoracoscopic lobectomy: a retrospective analysis and the influence of computed tomography-based

calcification assessment. J Thorac Cardiovasc Surg 2013;145:1512–8.
7. Endo S, Tsubochi H, Nakano T, et al. A dangerous venous variation in thoracoscopic right lower lobectomy. Ann Thorac Surg 2009;87:e9–10.
8. Asai K, Urabe N, Yajima K, et al. Right upper lobe venous drainage posterior to the bronchus intermedius: preoperative identification by computed tomography. Ann Thorac Surg 2005; 79:1866–71.
9. Marom EM, Herndon JE, Kim YH, et al. Variations in pulmonary venous drainage to the left atrium: implications for radiofrequency ablation. Radiology 2004;230:824–9.
10. Akiba T, Marushima H, Odaka M, et al. Pulmonary vein analysis using three-dimensional computed tomography angiography for thoracic surgery. Gen Thorac Cardiovasc Surg 2010;58:331–5.
11. Patel AG, Clark T, Oliver R, et al. Anomalous midline common ostium of the left and right inferior pulmonary veins: implications for pulmonary vein isolation in atrial fibrillation. Circ Arrhythm Electrophysiol 2008;1:407–8.
12. Shapiro M, Dodd JD, Brady TJ, et al. Common pulmonary venous ostium of the right and left inferior pulmonary veins: an unusual pulmonary vein anomaly depicted with 64-slice cardiac computed tomography. J Cardiovasc Electrophysiol 2007;18:110.
13. Akiba T, Marushima H, Morikawa T. Confirmation of a variant lingular vein anatomy during thoracoscopic surgery. Ann Thorac Cardiovasc Surg 2010;16:351–3.
14. Akiba T, Marushima H, Kamiya N, et al. Thoracoscopic lobectomy for treating cancer in a patient with an unusual vein anomaly. Ann Thorac Cardiovasc Surg 2011;17:501–3.
15. Sugimoto S, Izumiyama O, Yamashita A, et al. Anatomy of inferior pulmonary vein should be clarified in lower lobectomy. Ann Thorac Surg 1998;66: 1799–800.
16. Shiono H, Inoue A, Tomiyama N, et al. Safer video-assisted thoracoscopic thymectomy after location of thymic veins with multidetector computed tomography. Surg Endosc 2006;20:1419–22.
17. Hamid UI, Digney R, Soo L, et al. Incidence and outcome of re-entry injury in redo cardiac surgery: benefits of preoperative planning. Eur J Cardiothorac Surg 2014. http://dx.doi.org/10.1093/ejcts/ezu261.
18. Khan NU, Yonan N. Does preoperative computed tomography reduce the risks associated with re-do cardiac surgery? Interact Cardiovasc Thorac Surg 2009;9:119–23.
19. Saxena A, Chung SH, Ng A. Learning depth from single monocular images. Adv Neural Inf Process Syst 2005;18:1161.
20. Saxena A, Chung SH, Ng AY. 3-D depth reconstruction from a single still image. Int J Comput Vis 2008;76:53–69.
21. Jourdan IC, Dutson E, Garcia A, et al. Stereoscopic vision provides a significant advantage for precise robotic laparoscopy. Br J Surg 2004;91:879–85.
22. Das S, Ahuja N. Performance analysis of stereo, vergence, and focus as depth cues for active vision. IEEE Trans Pattern Analysis & machine Intelligence 1995;17:1213–9.
23. Lehmann KS, Ritz JP, Maass H, et al. A prospective, randomized study to test the transfer of basic psychomotor skills from virtual reality to physical reality in a comparable training setting. Ann Surg 2005;241:442–9.
24. Smith R, Day A, Rockall T, et al. Advanced stereoscopic projection technology significantly improves novice performance of minimally invasive surgical skills. Surg Endosc 2012;26:1522–7.
25. Chang L, Satava RM, Pellegrini CA, et al. Robotic surgery: identifying the learning curve through objective measurement of skill. Surg Endosc 2003;17:1744–8.
26. Camarillo DB, Krummel TM, Salisbury JK Jr. Robotic technology in surgery: past, present, and future. Am J Surg 2004;188:2S–15S.
27. Hernandez J, Bann S, Munz K, et al. Qualitative and quantitative analysis of the learning curve of a simulated task on the da Vinci system. Surg Endosc 2004;18:372–8.
28. Moorthy K, Munz Y, Dosis A, et al. Dexterity enhancement with robotic surgery. Surg Endosc 2004;18:790–5.
29. Demmy TL, James TA, Swanson SJ, et al. Troubleshooting video-assisted thoracic surgery lobectomy. Ann Thorac Surg 2005;79:1744–52 [discussion: 1753].
30. Berry MF, D'Amico TA. Complications of thoracoscopic pulmonary resection. Semin Thorac Cardiovasc Surg 2007;19:350–4.
31. Park BJ, Melfi F, Mussi A, et al. Robotic lobectomy for non-small cell lung cancer (NSCLC): long-term oncologic results. J Thorac Cardiovasc Surg 2012;143:383–9.
32. Hanna JM, Berry MF, D'Amico TA. Contraindications of video-assisted thoracoscopic surgical lobectomy and determinants of conversion to open. J Thorac Dis 2013;5:S182–9.
33. Cerfolio RJ, Bryant AS. How to teach robotic pulmonary resection. Semin Thorac Cardiovasc Surg 2013;25:76–82.
34. Xiao ZL, Mei JD, Pu Q, et al. Technical strategy for dealing with bleeding during thoracoscopic lung surgery. Ann Cardiothorac Surg 2014;3:213–5.
35. Puri V, Patel A, Majumder K, et al. Intraoperative conversion from video-assisted thoracoscopic surgery lobectomy to open thoracotomy: a study of

causes and implications. J Thorac Cardiovasc Surg 2015;149:55–62.
36. Lori Brown S, Woo EK. Surgical stapler-associated fatalities and adverse events reported to the Food and Drug Administration. J Am Coll Surg 2004; 199:374–81.
37. Kwazneski D, Six C, Stahlfeld K. The unacknowledged incidence of laparoscopic stapler malfunction. Surg Endosc 2013;27:86–9.
38. Yano M, Takao M, Fujinaga T, et al. Adverse events of pulmonary vascular stapling in thoracic surgery. Interact Cardiovasc Thorac Surg 2013;17:280–4.
39. Yim AP, Ho JK. Malfunctioning of vascular staple cutter during thoracoscopic lobectomy. J Thorac Cardiovasc Surg 1995;109:1252.
40. Craig SR, Walker WS. Potential complications of vascular stapling in thoracoscopic pulmonary resection. Ann Thorac Surg 1995;59:736–7 [discussion: 737–8].
41. Andonian S, Okeke Z, Okeke DA, et al. Device failures associated with patient injuries during robot-assisted laparoscopic surgeries: a comprehensive review of FDA MAUDE database. Can J Urol 2008; 15:3912–6.
42. Lucas SM, Pattison EA, Sundaram CP. Global robotic experience and the type of surgical system impact the types of robotic malfunctions and their clinical consequences: an FDA MAUDE review. BJU Int 2012;109:1222–7.
43. Friedman DC, Lendvay TS, Hannaford B. Instrument failures for the da Vinci surgical system: a Food and Drug Administration MAUDE database study. Surg Endosc 2013;27:1503–8.
44. Peterffy A, Henze A. Haemorrhagic complications during pulmonary resection. A retrospective review of 1428 resections with 113 haemorrhagic episodes. Scand J Thorac Cardiovasc Surg 1983;17: 283–7.
45. Kent M, Wang T, Whyte R, et al. Open, video-assisted thoracic surgery, and robotic lobectomy: review of a national database. Ann Thorac Surg 2014;97:236–44.
46. McKenna RJ, Houck W, Fuller CB. Video-assisted thoracic surgery lobectomy: experience with 1,100 cases. Ann Thorac Surg 2006;81:421–6.
47. Nakamura H. Systematic review of published studies on safety and efficacy of thoracoscopic and robot-assisted lobectomy for cancer. Ann Thorac Cardiovasc Surg 2014;20:93–8.
48. Swanson SJ, Miller DL, McKenna RJ, et al. Comparing robot-assisted surgical lobectomy with conventional video-assisted thoracic surgical lobectomy and wedge resection: results from a multihospital database (Premier). J Thorac Cardiovasc Surg 2014;147:929–37.
49. Cerfolio RJ, Bryant AS, Skyliard L, et al. Initial consecutive experience of completely portal robotic pulmonary resection with 4 arms. J Thorac Cardiovasc Surg 2011;142:740–6.
50. Flores RM, Ihekweazu U, Dycoco J, et al. Video-assisted thoracoscopic surgery (VATS) lobectomy: catastrophic intraoperative complications. J Thorac Cardiovasc Surg 2011;142:1412–7.
51. Augustin F, Schmid T, Bodner J. The robotic approach for mediastinal lesions. Int J Med Robot 2006;2:262–70.
52. Tovar EA. Pulmonary resection complicated by abrupt pericardial tamponade. Ann Thorac Surg 1995;60:1864.
53. McLean RH, Paradian BB, Nam MH. Pericardial tamponade: an unusual complication of lobectomy for lung cancer. Ann Thorac Surg 1999;67: 545–6.
54. Ozawa Y, Ichimura H, Sato T, et al. Cardiac tamponade due to coronary artery rupture after pulmonary resection. Ann Thorac Surg 2013;96:e97–9.
55. Chen J, Chen Z, Pang L, et al. A malformed staple causing cardiac tamponade after lobectomy. Ann Thorac Surg 2012;94:2107–8.
56. Dunning J, Walker WS. Pulmonary artery bleeding caused during VATS lobectomy. Ann Cardiothorac Surg 2012;1:109–10.
57. Lin MW, Lee JM, Lee YC. Penrose drain tube as a guide for endostaplers during lobectomy for endostaplers during lobectomy via video-assisted thoracoscopic surgery. Thorac Cardiovasc Surg 2010; 58:184–9.
58. Cerfolio RJ. Total port approach for robotic lobectomy. Thorac Surg Clin 2014;24:151–6.
59. Yamashita S, Tokuishi K, Moroga T, et al. Totally thoracoscopic surgery and troubleshooting for bleeding in non-small cell lung cancer. Ann Thorac Surg 2013;95:994–9.
60. Rendina EA, De Giacomo T, Venuta F, et al. Lung conservation techniques: bronchial sleeve resection and reconstruction of the pulmonary artery. Semin Surg Oncol 2000;18:165–72.
61. Watanabe A, Koyanagi T, Nakashima S, et al. How to clamp the main pulmonary artery during video-assisted thoracoscopic surgery lobectomy. Eur J Cardiothorac Surg 2007;31:129–31.
62. Kamiyoshihara M, Nagashima T, Ibe T, et al. A tip for controlling the main pulmonary artery during video-assisted thoracic major pulmonary resection: the outside-field vascular clamping technique. Interact Cardiovasc Thorac Surg 2010;11:693–5.
63. Nakanishi R, Oka S, Odate S. Video-assisted thoracic surgery major pulmonary resection requiring control of the main pulmonary artery. Interact Cardiovasc Thorac Surg 2009;994:618–22.
64. Nakanishi R, Yamashita T, Oka S. Initial experience of video-assisted thoracic surgery lobectomy with partial removal of the pulmonary artery. Interact Cardiovasc Thorac Surg 2008;7:996–1000.

65. Rendina EA, Venuta F, De Giacomo T, et al. Sleeve resection and prosthetic reconstruction of the pulmonary artery for lung cancer. Ann Thorac Surg 1999;68:995–1002.
66. Solli P, Spaggiari L, Grazia F, et al. Double prosthetic replacement of pulmonary artery and superior vena cava and sleeve lobectomy for lung cancer. Eur J Cardiothorac Surg 2001;20:1045–8.
67. Venuta F, Ciccone AM. Reconstruction of the pulmonary artery. Semin Thorac Cardiovasc Surg 2006;18:104–8.
68. Cerfolio RJ, Bryant AS. Surgical techniques and results for partial or circumferential sleeve resection of the pulmonary artery for patients with on-small cell lung cancer. Ann Thorac Surg 2007;83:1971–7.
69. Ibrahim M, Maurizi G, Venuta F, et al. Reconstruction of the bronchus and pulmonary artery. Thorac Surg Clin 2013;23:337–47.
70. Endo T, Tetsuka K, Yamamoto S, et al. Transection of left common pulmonary vein during left upper lobectomy: how should it be reconstructed. J Surg Case Rep 2012;(12). http://dx.doi.org/10.1093/jscr/rjs030.
71. Nakamura T, Koide M, Nakamura H, et al. The common trunk of the left pulmonary vein injured incidentally during lung cancer surgery. Ann Thorac Surg 2009;87:954–5.
72. Yu DP, Han Y, Zhao QY, et al. Pulmonary lobectomy combined with pulmonary arterioplasty by complete video-assisted thoracic surgery in patients with lung cancer. Asian Pac J Cancer Prev 2013; 14:6061–4.
73. Han Y, Zhou S, Yu D, et al. Video-assisted thoracic surgery (VATS) left upper sleeve lobectomy with partial pulmonary artery resection. J Thorac Dis 2013;5:S301–3.
74. Jones RO, Casali G, Walker WS. Does failed video-assisted lobectomy for lung cancer prejudice immediate and long-term outcomes? Ann Thorac Surg 2008;86:235–9.
75. Park JS, Kim HK, Choi YS, et al. Unplanned conversion to thoracotomy during video-assisted thoracic surgery lobectomy does not compromise the surgical outcome. World J Surg 2011;35:590–5.
76. Sawada S, Komori E, Yamashita M. Evaluation of video-assisted thoracoscopic surgery lobectomy requiring emergency conversion to thoracotomy. Eur J Cardiothorac Surg 2009;36:487–90.
77. Rusch VW. Extrapleural pneumonectomy and extended pleurectomy/decortication for malignant pleural mesothelioma: the Memorial Sloan Kettering Cancer Center approach. Ann Cardiothorac Surg 2012;1:523–31.
78. Zellos L, Jaklitsch MT, Bueno R, et al. Treatment of malignant mesothelioma: extrapleural pneumonectomy with intraoperative chemotherapy. J Thorac Cardiovasc Surg 2009;138:405–11.
79. Rai SP, Kaul SK, Tripathi RK, et al. Decortication in chronic pleural empyema. Lung India 2006;23:100–2.
80. Masaoka A, Yamakawa Y, Niwa H, et al. Extended thymectomy for myasthenia gravis patients: a 20-year review. Ann Thorac Surg 1996;62:853–9.
81. Kattach H, Anastasiadis K, Cleuziou J, et al. Transsternal thymectomy for myasthenia gravis: surgical outcome. Ann Thorac Surg 2006;81:305–8.
82. Shrager JB, Nathan D, Brinster C, et al. Outcomes after 151 extended transcervical thymectomies for myasthenia gravis. Ann Thorac Surg 2006;82:1863–9.
83. Shrager JB. Extended transcervical thymectomy: the ultimate minimally invasive approach. Ann Thorac Surg 2010;89:S2128–34.
84. Roviaro G, Varoli F, Nucca O, et al. Videothoracoscopic approach to primary mediastinal pathology. Chest 2000;117:1179–83.
85. Whitson BA, Andrade RS, Mitiek MO, et al. Thoracoscopic thymectomy: technical pearls to a 21st century approach. J Thorac Dis 2013;5:129–34.
86. Soon JL, Agasthian T. Harmonic scalpel in video-assisted thoracoscopic thymic resections. Asian Cardiovasc Thorac Ann 2008;16:366–9.
87. Ashbaugh DG. Mediastinoscopy. Arch Surg 1970; 100:568–73.
88. Cybulshky IJ, Bennet WF. Mediastinoscopy as a routine outpatient procedure. Ann Thorac Surg 1994;58:176–8.
89. Urschel JD. Conservative management (packing) of hemorrhage complicating mediastinoscopy. Ann Thorac Cardiovasc Surg 2000;6:9–12.
90. Park BJ, Flores R, Downey RJ, et al. Management of major hemorrhage during mediastinoscopy. J Thorac Cardiovasc Surg 2003;126:726–31.
91. Lemaire A, Nikolic I, Petersen T, et al. Nine-year single center experience with cervical mediastinoscopy: complications and false negative rate. Ann Thorac Surg 2006;82:1185–90.
92. Hammoud ZT, Anderson RC, Meyers BF, et al. The current role of mediastinoscopy in the evaluation of thoracic disease. J Thorac Cardiovasc Surg 1999; 118:894–9.
93. De Waele M, Serra-Mitjans M, Hendriks J, et al. Accuracy and survival of repeat mediastinoscopy after induction therapy for non-small cell lung cancer in a combined series of 104 patients. Eur J Cardiothorac Surg 2008;33:824–8.
94. Lardinois D, Schallberger A, Betticher D, et al. Postinduction video-mediastinoscopy is as accurate and safe as videomediastinoscopy in patients without pretreatment for potentially operable nonsmall-cell lung cancer. Ann Thorac Surg 2003; 75:1102–6.
95. Stamatis G, Fechner S, Hillejan L, et al. Repeat mediastinoscopy as a restaging procedure. Pneumologie 2005;59:862–6.

96. Louie BE, Kapur S, Farivar AS, et al. Safety and utility of mediastinoscopy in non-small cell lung cancer in a complex mediastinum. Ann Thorac Surg 2011;92:278–83.
97. Jaus M, Macchiarini P. Superior vena cava and innominate vein reconstruction in thoracic malignancies: cryopreserved graft reconstruction. Semin Thorac Cardiovasc Surg 2011;23:330–5.
98. Dartevelle PG, Chapelier AR, Pastorino U, et al. Long-term follow-up after prosthetic replacement of the superior vena cava combined with resection of mediastinal-pulmonary malignant tumors. J Thorac Cardiovasc Surg 1991;102:259–65.
99. Spaggiari L, Leo F, Veronesi G, et al. Superior vena cava resection for lung and mediastinal malignancies: a single-center experience with 70 cases. Ann Thorac Surg 2007;83:223–30.
100. Okereke IC, Kesler KA. Superior vena cava and innominate vein reconstruction in thoracic malignancies: single-vein reconstruction. Semin Thorac Cardiovasc Surg 2011;23:323–5.
101. Odell DD, Liao K. Superior vena cava and innominate vein reconstruction in thoracic malignancies: double-vein reconstruction. Semin Thorac Cardiovasc Surg 2011;23:326–9.
102. Shintani Y, Ohta M, Minami M, et al. Long-term patency after replacement of the brachiocephalic veins combined with resection of mediastinal tumors. J Thorac Cardiovasc Surg 2005;129:809–12.
103. Witte B, Wolf M, Hillebrand H, et al. Extended cervical mediastinoscopy revisited. Eur J Cardiothorac Surg 2014;4:114–9.
104. Johnston RH Jr, Wall MJ Jr, Mattox KL. Innominate artery trauma: a thirty-year experience. J Vasc Surg 1993;17(1):134–9.
105. Smith SJ, Lyons OT, Patel AS, et al. Endovascular repair of the aorta and aortic arch arteries damaged during mediastinoscopy. J Vasc Surg 2012;55:138–40.
106. Wall MJ, Mattox KL, DeBakey ME. Injuries to the azygous venous system. J Trauma 2006;60:357–62.
107. Baigrie RJ, Watson DI, Game PA, et al. Vascular perils during laparoscopic dissection of the esophageal hiatus. Br J Surg 1997;84:556–7.
108. Leggett PL, Bissell CD, Churchman-Winn R. Aortic injury during laparoscopic fundoplication: an underreported complication. Surg Endosc 2002;16:362.
109. Yano F, Omura N, Tsuboi K, et al. Thoracic aortic injury during laparoscopic fundoplication for reflux esophagitis. Int J Surg 2008;6(6):490–2.
110. Bonavina L, Bona D, Saino G, et al. Injury of the thoracic aorta during laparoscopic esophagectomy. Surg Laparosc Endosc Percutan Tech 2009;19:e55–6.
111. Nagpal AP, Soni H, Haribhakti SP. Left hepatic vein injury during laparoscopic antireflux surgery for large para-oesophageal hiatus hernia. J Minim Access Surg 2009;5:72–4.
112. Orringer MB, Marshall B, Chang AC, et al. Two thousand transhiatal esophagectomies: changing trends, lessons learned. Ann Surg 2007;246:363–74.
113. Javed A, Pal S, Chaubal GN, et al. Management and outcome of intrathoracic bleeding due to vascular injury during transhiatal esophagectomy. J Gastrointest Surg 2011;15:262–6.
114. Pantvaidya GH, Mistry RC, Ghanekar VR, et al. Injury of an aberrant subclavian artery: a rare complication of video assisted thoracoscopic esophagectomy. Ann Thorac Cardiovasc Surg 2005;11:35–7.
115. Weissenbacher A, Bodner J. Robotic surgery of the mediastinum. Thorac Surg Clin 2010;20:331–9.
116. van Hillegersberg R, Boone J, Draaisma WA, et al. First experience with robot-assisted thoracoscopic esophagolymphadenectomy for esophageal cancer. Surg Endosc 2006;20:1435–9.
117. Luketich JD, Pennathur A, Awais O, et al. Outcomes after minimally invasive esophagectomy: review of over 1000 patients. Ann Surg 2012;256:95–103.
118. Schieman C, Wigle DA, Deschamps C, et al. Patterns of operative mortality following esophagectomy. Dis Esophagus 2012;25:645–51.
119. Ponten JE, van der Horst S, Nieuwenhuijzen GA, et al. Early severe mediastinal bleeding after esophagectomy: a potentially lethal complication. J Thorac Dis 2013;5:E58–60.
120. Ahn M, Shin BS, Park MH. Aortoesophageal fistula secondary to placement of an esophageal stent: emergent treatment with cyanoacrylate and endovascular stent graft. Ann Vasc Surg 2010;24:555.e1–5.
121. Whitelocke D, Maddaus M, Andrade R, et al. Gastroaortic fistula: a rare and lethal complication of esophageal stenting after esophagectomy. J Thorac Cardiovasc Surg 2010;140:e49–50.
122. Schweigert M, Dubecz A, Stadhuber RJ, et al. Risk of stent-related aortic erosion after endoscopic stent insertion for intrathoracic anastomotic leaks after esophagectomy. Ann Thorac Surg 2011;92:513–8.
123. Ikeda Y, Morita N, Kurihara H, et al. A primary aortoesophageal fistula due to esophageal carcinoma successfully treated with endoluminal aortic stent grafting. J Thorac Cardiovasc Surg 2006;131:486–7.
124. Kato N, Tadanori H, Tanaka K, et al. Aortoesophageal fistula relief of massive hematemesis with an endovascular stent-graft. Eur J Radiol 2000;34:63–6.
125. Okita R, Mukaida H, Takiyama W, et al. Successful surgical treatment of aortoesophageal fistula after esophagectomy. Ann Thorac Surg 2005;79:1059–61.

126. Mok VW, Ting AC, Law S, et al. Combined endovascular stent grafting and endoscopic injection of fibrin sealant for aortoenteric fistula complicating esophagectomy. J Vasc Surg 2004;40:1234–7.
127. Matono S, Fujita H, Tanaka T, et al. Thoracic endovascular aortic repair for aortic complications after esophagectomy. Dis Esophagus 2011;24:E36–40.
128. Firbes TL, Harding GE. Endovascular repair of salmonella infected abdominal aortic aneurysm: a word of caution. J Vasc Surg 2006;44:198–200.
129. Kan CD, Lee HL, Yang YJ. Outcome after endovascular stent graft treatment for mycotic aortic aneurysm: a systemic review. J Vasc Surg 2007;46:906–12.
130. Chandler J, Corson S, Way L. Three spectra of laparoscopic entry access injuries. J Am Coll Surg 2001;192:478–91.
131. Gregg RO. Aortic compressor. Am J Surg 1966; 111:609.
132. DeBakey ME, Creech O Jr, Morris GC Jr. Aneurysm of thoracoabdominal aorta involving the celiac, superior mesenteric and renal arteries. Report of four cases treated by resection and homograft replacement. Ann Surg 1956;144:549.
133. Elkins RC, DeMeester TR, Brawley RK. Surgical exposure of the upper abdominal aorta and its branches. Surgery 1970;70:622–7.
134. Joyce WP, Ward AS. Supraceliac clamping: an underused alternative in aortic surgery. Ann Vasc Surg 1990;4:393–6.
135. Yau P, Watson DI, Devitt PG, et al. Early reoperation following laparoscopic antireflux surgery. Am J Surg 2000;179:172–6.
136. Kyriazanos ID, Tachibana M, Yoshimura H, et al. Impact of splenectomy on the early outcome after oesophagectomy for squamous cell carcinoma of the oesophagus. Eur J Surg Oncol 2002;28:113–9.
137. Gockel I, Kneist W, Junginger T. Influence of splenectomy on perioperative morbidity and long-term survival after esophagectomy in patients with esophageal carcinoma. Dis Esophagus 2005;18:311–5.
138. Black E, Niamat J, Boddu S, et al. Unplanned splenectomy during oesophagectomy does not affect survival. Eur J Cardiothorac Surg 2006; 29:244–7.
139. Deng YJ, Rong TH, Zhang LJ, et al. Influence of unexpected simultaneous splenectomy on postoperative complications and prognosis of patients undergoing radical esophagectomy for esophageal carcinoma. Ai Zheng 2007;26:983–6.
140. Aminian A, Mirsharifi R, Karimian F, et al. Influence of splenectomy on morbidity of esophageal cancer surgery. Scand J Surg 2010;99:9–13.
141. Leemans R, Manson W, Snijder JA, et al. Immune response capacity after human splenic autotransplantation: restoration of response to individual pneumococcal vaccine subtypes. Ann Surg 1999; 229:279–85.

Endotracheal Tube Management and Obstructed Airway

Manu Sancheti, MD[a], Seth Force, MD[b,*]

KEYWORDS

• Anesthesia • Lung isolation • Airway obstruction • One-lung ventilation • Rigid bronchoscopy

KEY POINTS

- While managing the surgical procedure, the surgeon should be constantly aware of the respiratory mechanics and control of the airway via the endotracheal tube.
- Operations in the pleural cavity usually necessitate lung isolation.
- The surgeon and anesthesiologist should have a clear plan in terms of a strategy for intubation, a management algorithm for respiratory problems, and an established crisis protocol.
- Proper management of an acute central airway obstruction requires a thorough knowledge of anatomy and techniques, rapid decision making, and an intimate communication with a skilled anesthesiologist.
- The surgeon must be aware of multiple ventilation strategies including standard ventilation, jet ventilation, and, if necessary, extracorporeal membrane oxygenation (ECMO) if intubation is not possible.
- Surgeons must also be aware of multiple intubation strategies including standard intubation, double-lumen tube intubation, laryngeal mask airway, cross-field ventilation, and rigid bronchoscopy.
- Rigid bronchoscopic management is the most efficient initial step in the management of a central airway obstruction.

INTRODUCTION

The scope of general thoracic surgery encompasses a wide array of procedures and corresponding anesthetic techniques. Thoracic anesthesia is a field requiring mastery of pulmonary anatomy and physiology, as well as technical prowess in the stabilization of an adequate airway through various modalities. In addition, in most cases, patients undergoing thoracic surgery include those with difficult airways and significant respiratory pathologies, thus increasing the complexity of the anesthesiologist's role. Finally, the thoracic surgical procedure usually involves entry into the pleural cavity, thereby necessitating lung isolation techniques.

The general thoracic surgeon is not spared from these complexities. While managing the surgical procedure, the surgeon should be constantly aware of the respiratory mechanics and control of the airway via the endotracheal tube. The surgeon should be familiar with the various

The authors have nothing to disclose.

[a] Division of Cardiothoracic Surgery, Emory St. Joseph's Hospital, Emory University School of Medicine, 5665 Peachtree Dunwoody Road, Suite 200, Atlanta, GA 30342, USA; [b] General Thoracic Surgery, Division of Cardiothoracic Surgery, Emory University Hospital, Emory University School of Medicine, 1365A Clifton Road Northeast, Atlanta, GA 30322, USA

* Corresponding author.
E-mail address: sforce@emory.edu

Thorac Surg Clin 25 (2015) 279–288
http://dx.doi.org/10.1016/j.thorsurg.2015.04.002
1547-4127/15/$ – see front matter Published by Elsevier Inc.

techniques of airway management and lung isolation. Also, the surgeon and anesthesiologist should have knowledge of the potential catastrophes and be able to communicate proper crisis protocol plans. The following sections detail the surgeon's role in managing the airway and endotracheal tube by explaining intraoperative respiratory monitoring, techniques of lung isolation, and potential complications therein.

MONITORING

Accurate respiratory monitoring is vital to good outcomes. Modern anesthesia ventilators provide real-time data regarding pressure-volume relationships in the ventilated lungs. Changes in pressure may be issues related to the anesthesia circuit or the lung parenchyma and airway itself, such as an obstructed airway or auto–positive end-expiratory pressure. Similarly, changes in tidal volume (inspiratory and expiratory) can relate to the patient's baseline pulmonary function or be secondary to the operative procedure, that is, air leaks. The intricacies of ventilation strategies are beyond the scope of this article; however, it is important to understand that a working knowledge of these details is necessary.

In the diseased lungs that are often managed in thoracic surgery, gas exchange is an important variable to closely monitor. Hypoxemia (arterial saturation <90%) is especially prevalent in lung isolation techniques. Fortunately, with improved modalities in the past 25 years, the incidence of intraoperative hypoxemia has dropped from 25% to 1% in thoracic surgery.[1] The intraoperative measurement of oxygenation is done by pulse oximetry and arterial blood gases. Advances in technology have yielded reliable pulse oximeters so that ventilation management decisions can be made based on their measurements; this permits decreased arterial blood gas requirements without a sacrifice in outcomes.[2] However, it has been shown that pulse oximetry has a slower rate of change when compared with arterial saturation. Also, pulse oximetry measurement usually provides a lower reading than a simultaneous arterial blood gas.[3] Continuous blood gas monitoring devices have been developed but are not yet in widespread use.[4] Therefore, it is recommended to use continuous pulse oximetry with intermittent arterial blood gas measurements as an adjunct. Finally, the measurement of cerebral oximetry may have utility; however, the usefulness of the data in thoracic surgery has yet to be defined.[5]

Carbon dioxide monitoring in patients undergoing thoracic surgery is as important as oxygenation. Hypocarbia or hypercarbia are signs of significant ventilation dysfunction. Similar to oxygenation monitoring, different modalities are available with different advantages and disadvantages. Arterial blood gas measurements usually provide the most accurate result, but require more time and frequent blood draws; their usefulness seems to be best in an intermittent role. At the time of intubation, end-tidal CO_2 has been shown to be an excellent determinant of successful endotracheal intubation.[6] In terms of continuous monitoring, both transcutaneous and end-tidal carbon dioxide monitoring are currently used. Studies have shown that in thoracic surgery procedures, especially those requiring 1-lung ventilation, transcutaneous carbon dioxide monitoring provides more accurate results than end-tidal carbon dioxide.[7]

LUNG ISOLATION

A unique aspect of operations in the pleural cavity is the necessity for lung isolation and 1-lung ventilation. One-lung ventilation permits the following:

- Improved surgical exposure
- Prevention of contamination of contralateral lung
- Airway control in bronchopleural fistula, sleeve resection, or pneumonectomy
- Differential lung ventilation

Successful methods to perform lung isolation and 1-lung ventilation have been available since the introduction of red rubber double-lumen endotracheal tube (DLT) by Björk and Carlens[8] in 1950. Although other techniques do exist for certain circumstances, the primary methods used to provide lung isolation include the DLT and bronchial blockade. Advantages of both modalities are listed in **Table 1**. Although each method has its own pros and cons, the general consensus remains that the thoracic anesthesiologist and surgeon should be facile in the use of a variety of techniques based on the patient's specific situation.[9]

Double-Lumen Endotracheal Tube

A DLT consists of tubes bonded together side by side, with an endotracheal component and an endobronchial component and each lumen intended to ventilate 1 lung. DLTs are made as left- and right-sided tubes. Left-sided tubes are more commonly used because of the relative ease of positioning the bronchial tube component in the longer left main bronchus. Right-sided DLTs must be precisely placed into the right main stem bronchus so that the ventilation opening for the right upper lobe is placed over the upper lobe

Table 1
Advantages of DLT and bronchial blocker

DLT	Bronchial Blocker
Allows suctioning of secretions and blood	Less traumatic to airway
Easy conversion from 1-lung ventilation to 2-lung ventilation	Wide variety of products and sizes
Allows absolute lung separation (ie, bleeding, pus, total lung lavage)	Allows selective lobar blockade
Faster placement	Useful for patients with tracheostomy or abnormal bronchial anatomy
Faster lung collapse	Can be used through standard endotracheal tube for patients with difficult airway or on prolonged mechanical ventilation
Less-frequent malposition	—

bronchial orifice to allow for upper lobe ventilation. Indications for a right-sided DLT are shown in **Box 1**. All DLTs have an endobronchial cuff, which allows separate ventilation of the right and left lungs. The DLT also has an endotracheal cuff, which seals both lungs from the environment, similar to that on a single-lumen endotracheal tube.

Although DLTs provide excellent lung isolation, their placement can be somewhat cumbersome as opposed to that of the single-lumen endotracheal tube. First, identifying the proper size of endotracheal tube is vital. General guidelines state using a 41F DLT for men and a 35F to 37F DLT for women.[10] However, a tube that is too large could risk damage to the bronchial tree, whereas a small tube is more susceptible to slipping out of position. In general, the bronchial tip of the DLT should be 1 to 2 mm smaller than the diameter of the distal bronchus.[11] Several methods have been suggested to estimate the appropriate DLT:

- If the tube passes the glottis without difficulty, it is estimated to not be oversized for the main bronchus.[9]
- The tracheal diameter at clavicles can be measured on preoperative posterior-anterior chest radiograph.[12]
- The left main bronchus can be measured on preoperative computed tomographic scan.[13]
- Measurements can be made from 3-dimensional reconstructions of tracheobronchial anatomy.[14]

The next challenge for DLT use is appropriate placement. Two primary methods have been proposed: blind placement and fiber-optic-bronchoscopy-assisted placement. Blind placement entails standard insertion of the endotracheal tube with direct laryngoscopy, followed by a 90° counterclockwise turn to the side of the appropriate DLT. The tube is advanced to resistance or 29 cm.[15] Of note, blind placement alone has been shown to have a malposition rate up to 30%.[16] Fiber-optic bronchoscopy can therefore be used as an adjunct to confirm appropriate location during initial placement as well as when the patient is fully positioned in lateral decubitus.

Intraoperative complications of DLT likely result from poor sizing, malposition, and airway trauma. Malposition can obviously lead to changes in pulmonary mechanics and gas exchange. Also, surgical exposure can be hindered, possibly at an unsafe point in the operation. Malposition of an undersized DLT too distal in a lobar bronchus can lead to significant barotrauma and subsequent tension pneumothorax.[17] Airway trauma can also occur because of injury of the membranous trachea with insertion or manipulation of DLT. This trauma can present as loss of tidal volume (air leak), subcutaneous emphysema, bleeding, or protrusion of DLT into surgical field.[11] Management of these emergencies should include control of airway, fiber-optic bronchoscopy for diagnosis, and definitive surgical repair. In most cases, the DLT can be retracted to the appropriate position and away from the site injury, thus

Box 1
Indications for right-sided DLT

Left sleeve resection

Left pneumonectomy

Left tracheobronchial injury

Left single-lung transplantation

Tumor involvement or compression at left main stem bronchus

Descending thoracic aortic aneurysm

allowing lung isolation and exposure for definitive airway repair. Rare reports have been described requiring the extension of the iatrogenic bronchotomy and cross-table ventilation through the site.[18]

Specific clinical situations in which lung isolation by DLT intubation is invaluable involve bronchopleural and tracheoesophageal fistulas; this includes both perioperative and long-term mechanical ventilation airway management. The key component in these difficult patients entails the isolation of the fistulous opening from continued ventilation. Owing to the low resistance to airflow, ventilation preferentially moves through the fistula. This movement of ventilation results in hypoventilation of the lungs, tension pneumothorax, and persistence, if not worsening, of the fistula.[19] In addition, in the case of tracheoesophageal fistula, ventilation through the tract can lead to esophageal and gastric distension. Finally, fluid can drain from the affected hemithorax through the fistula into the normal hemithorax, especially in cases in which the patient is placed in the lateral decubitus position.[20]

Important clinical strategies in these challenging scenarios include the following:

- Placement of chest tube on affected side before any intervention.
- Esophageal and gastric decompression via nasogastric tube before intervention.
- DLT placement under bronchoscopic guidance to ensure correct placement and relation of tube to fistula.
- Placement of right-sided DLT, especially in left-sided fistulas.
- Prompt clamping of lumen ventilating the lung ipsilateral to fistula.
- Confirmation of appropriate placement with bronchoscopy before lateral decubitus positioning.

Bronchial Blocker

The endobronchial blocker is an alternative method to lung isolation that is composed of blockade of the main stem bronchus or lobar bronchus to allow lung collapse distal to the site of occlusion.[21] Many devices are available and are primarily used within a single-lumen endotracheal tube. Although this article does not detail the specifics of each blocker, the general premise of placement includes bronchoscopic guidance of the blocker into the appropriate main stem or lobar bronchus. Although the bronchial blocker can be used in any situation in which lung isolation is needed, it is especially advantageous over a DLT in specific situations. These situations are

- Tracheostomy
- Lobar blockade
- Difficult airway
- Anatomic abnormalities
- Requirement of postoperative mechanical ventilation

The primary complication related to bronchial blocker involves malposition of the blocker itself with subsequent loss of lung isolation. This scenario is an especially prevalent and bothersome one in right upper lobe operations because of the proximal takeoff of the right upper lobe bronchus.[22] Bauer and colleagues[23] showed that bronchial blockers had a higher frequency of malposition when compared with DLT in thoracoscopy. Interestingly, bronchial blockers have been demonstrated to take an average of 30 seconds to 1 minute longer for appropriate placement by a cardiothoracic anesthesiologist. The same study showed that bronchial blockers more likely require assisted suction to fully deflate the isolated lung and that the rate of deflation was slower. Most importantly, however, no change was noted in surgical exposure between the 2 modalities.[24]

Adjunct Ventilation Modalities

DLT intubation and bronchial blocker placement are effective in providing lung isolation in the vast majority of cases requiring 1-lung ventilation. However, situations (**Box 2**) do arise in which these isolation techniques are not efficacious. Consequently, a wide array of adjunct modalities have been developed to provide the means necessary to perform the definitive surgical procedure without sacrificing patient safety. Some of these modalities include

Box 2
Clinical scenarios for adjunct ventilation strategies

Tracheostomy or permanent tracheal stoma

Difficult airway/inability to convert single-lumen endotracheal tube

Morbid obesity

Postlaryngectomy

History of head and neck radiation

Congenital craniofacial abnormalities

Airway anatomic abnormalities

Prior contralateral lung resection

Inability to ventilate/oxygenate with 1-lung ventilation

- Regional/local anesthesia
- Selective lobar collapse
- Intermittent ipsilateral lung ventilation
- High-frequency positive-pressure or jet ventilation of the ipsilateral lung
- Single-lumen endotracheal tube placement into ipsilateral main stem bronchus
- Single-lumen endotracheal tube intubation with low tidal volume ventilation[25]
- Single-lumen endotracheal tube intubation and carbon dioxide insufflation[26]
- Cross-table ventilation via surgical bronchotomy or tracheotomy[27]
- Cardiopulmonary support (cardiopulmonary bypass, extracorporeal membrane oxygenator)

SUMMARY

Thoracic surgery encompasses a wide array of surgical techniques, most of which require lung isolation for surgical exposure in the pleural cavity; this, in turn, demands an excellent knowledge of respiratory mechanics and modalities of airway control. Most importantly, a clear plan should exist between the surgeon and anesthesiologist in terms of the planned treatment algorithm, as well as concise escape plans for potential crises.

OBSTRUCTED AIRWAY

Introduction

Of the various types of intraoperative crises, management of the acute critical central airway obstruction can often be the most demanding on the thoracic surgeon. Proper management involves a thorough knowledge of anatomy and techniques, rapid decision making, and an intimate communication with a skilled anesthesiologist. The obstruction can be a life-threatening emergency requiring prompt treatment to avoid significant hypoxia or death.[28] The location of the obstruction dictates the appropriate treatment algorithm. An upper airway obstruction is defined as from the oronasal passages to the glottis.[29] Securing an airway distal to this proximal obstruction is the appropriate initial management and beyond the scope of this article. This section focuses on the management of central airway obstruction defined as from the subglottic space to the level of the lobar bronchi orifices.

Presentation

The clinical presentation of acute central airway obstruction can be varied and nonspecific. Possible signs and symptoms include

- Dyspnea
- Cough
- Stridor/wheezing
- Hoarseness
- Orthopnea
- Postobstructive pneumonia
- Hypoxia

Cause

The cause of central airway obstruction can be equally varied, with a myriad of potential causes, both malignant and nonmalignant (**Box 3**). Direct extension is the most common cause of malignant airway obstruction; this most likely represents a bronchogenic carcinoma, rather than primary tracheal carcinomas, which are exceedingly rare with an incidence of about 700 cases per year in the United States.[30] Esophageal tumors, thyroid tumors, thymic carcinomas, or other mediastinal tumors also have the potential to extend into the trachea. Malignant airway obstructions distal to the carina are most likely because of carcinoid tumors.[31] In terms of nonmalignant central airway obstructions, the most likely cause includes tracheal stenosis secondary to postintubation or posttracheostomy injury.[32]

Anesthesia

Careful anesthetic management in the evaluation and treatment of central airway obstruction is a point of distinct emphasis.[33] As mentioned previously, clear communication between the surgeon and an experienced anesthesiologist is a key principle. The surgeon should be present and involved during induction, with all necessary operative

Box 3
Causes of central airway obstruction

Malignant primary airway tumor

Benign primary airway tumor

Extrathoracic disease metastatic to airway

Adjacent tumor extending into airway (lung, esophagus)

Mediastinal tumor

Sarcoidosis

Infectious lymphadenopathy

Tracheomalacia

Bronchial webs

Postintubation stricture

Granulation tissue

Vascular sling or aneurysm

Inspissated secretions/blood

equipment available. It is important that the surgeon develop an efficient emergency airway plan before induction. Tracheostomy or cricothyroidotomy may not be adequate in patients with central airway obstructions, and therefore, the goal is to obtain a secure airway that traverses the obstruction or originates at a point distal to the obstruction to provide ventilation to the distal bronchial tree. It is a vital tenet that the anesthesiologist avoid paralytic agents until the surgeon has obtained a secure airway; this prevents the dire situation of the combination of airway obstruction and apnea. Standard preoxygenation with 100% oxygen is administered followed by induction with inhalation agents, such as halothane or sevoflurane.[33] This procedure allows the patient to maintain spontaneous respirations during induction as well as quicker resumption of spontaneous respirations at the conclusion of the procedure. Corticosteroids should be administered (dexamethasone 4–10 mg every 6 h for 24 h) to lessen traumatic edema. Some investigators suggest ventilating with the rigid bronchoscope or placement of an endotracheal tube until the patient is fully awake before extubation.[34] Rarely, complex techniques, such as transtracheal jet ventilation, cardiopulmonary bypass, or ECMO, may be necessary to allow safe establishment of a secure airway before the definitive procedure. Lang and colleagues[35] have shown favorable results with the use of venoarterial ECMO in their patients undergoing complex tracheobronchial or carinal resection.

Management

Owing to the tenuous nature of the patient's airway with a central airway obstruction, a well-defined treatment algorithm must be in place before any planned intervention. Definitive surgical resection and reconstruction is the therapy of choice for central airway obstruction.[36] However, the feasibility of this approach for acute central airway obstruction is extremely rare.[37] Therefore, bronchoscopic management is the most efficient initial step in the management of a central airway obstruction.[38] Ost and colleagues[39] showed a 93% success rate of therapeutic bronchoscopy in reopening the airway to 50% of normal. This technique allows effective diagnosis with the potential of curative intent while allowing for a stable airway.

Rigid instrumentation provides the best means to diagnose and treat an airway obstruction. The rigid scope can stent the airway open and allow for ventilation, while also allowing passage of the flexible bronchoscope to visualize and inspect the airway. A ventilating rigid bronchoscope ranging from pediatric to adult sizes should be available. Airway management via the rigid bronchoscope uses both standard and jet ventilation techniques. Standard ventilation with a routine anesthesia circuit can be performed by the placement of a small endotracheal tube (ETT) in the rigid bronchoscope, or in most cases, the attachment of the circuit to a designated area on the rigid bronchoscope itself. Similarly, jet ventilation can be provided by the jet ventilator tubing within the bronchoscope or attached to an adaptor on the bronchoscope. Jet ventilation is associated with higher incidences of barotrauma, hypercarbia, and hypoxia compared with standard ventilation. Importantly, ventilation through the bronchoscope is limited by inadequate seal of the airway; this can be improved with cricoid pressure or occlusion of the upper airway with gauze or the surgeon's hand.

The rounded tips of the rigid bronchoscope allows for easier maneuvering under the epiglottis and past areas of tight obstruction. The initial goals of rigid bronchoscopy for central airway obstruction are to secure a proper airway and relief of the obstruction. To accomplish the latter, the characteristics of the obstruction should be carefully examined to better delineate the appropriate treatment algorithm. In general, postintubation or posttraumatic cicatricial stenosis can be dilated. Malignant airway obstructions require recanalization, whereas extrinsic compressive obstructions can be stented. These methods offer a stable, patent airway to defer until definitive treatment is used. The following sections detail the emergent management of central airway obstruction.

Dilation

Cicatricial stenoses are most amenable to endoscopic dilation as a bridge to definitive surgical resection or, occasionally, as the definitive procedure itself. However, the primary goal should always be the stabilization of a secure airway. Postintubation stenosis is the most common nonmalignant cause of central airway obstruction, followed by idiopathic, posttraumatic, postirradiation, and inflammatory causes. In most cases, emergent management of these stenoses require placement of a ventilating rigid bronchoscope followed by serial dilations with increasing scope sizes. However, if the stenosis were at the site of a former tracheostomy stoma, emergent airway stabilization would be best achieved with the placement of a tracheostomy at the site of the stoma/stenosis; this is because of the complex nature of stomal stenosis that often renders it resistant to endoscopic dilation in that the stenosis immediately reoccurs after removal of the rigid bronchoscope.

Standard endoscopic dilation involves various sizes of pediatric and adult rigid bronchoscopes. Based on the diameter of the stenosis, the smallest passable rigid bronchoscope is maneuvered across the stenosis in a corkscrewing motion without using excessive force that may damage the membranous trachea. The patient is ventilated via the rigid bronchoscope until it is deemed safe by the anesthesiologist to remove the scope and replace with the next larger size. Sequential dilations up to 8 mm should be performed at which point one would be confident in the caliber of the airway for adequate airflow. The following adjuncts to this method have been described:

- Use of 14-mm tracheoscope placed just distal to the vocal cords through which sequential rigid bronchoscopes are passed.
- Use of sequential semirigid esophageal dilators through tracheoscope or rigid bronchoscope.[40]
- Use of Savary esophageal dilators (Wilson-Cook, USA) with flexible bronchoscopic guidance and fluoroscopy.[41]
- Use of balloon dilation.[42,43]

These methods can provide several weeks to months of airway stability and symptom control, which allows a time interval for appropriate careful evaluation and preparation for the definitive surgical procedure. In certain instances, serial dilations can maintain an adequate quality of life and control of symptoms for some patients. Serial dilations may be specifically pertinent to patients with nonreconstructable lesions.

Recanalization

Endobronchial complications have been noted in up to 30% of newly diagnosed lung cancer in the United States.[44] The emergent management of an obstructing central airway tumor must be removal to provide recanalization of the airway for spontaneous breathing. Effective tumor removal is performed with the rigid bronchoscope with the addition of biopsy devices and suction. The rounded tip of the bronchoscope can also be used to core out the tumor. The rigid bronchoscope can also be carefully maneuvered past the obstructing tumor to allow ventilation to the postobstruction airways. Finally, because of the hypervascularity of many of these tumors, the rigid bronchoscope provides the means to control bleeding with several adjuncts, such as direct pressure, laser treatment, cryotherapy, and electrocautery. Importantly, the fraction of inspired oxygen should be maintained less than 50% to lessen the potential for intraoperative airway fires.[45] When a fire does occur, the patient must be immediately disconnected from the anesthesia circuit and the fire extinguished using wet gauze and/or saline. The ETT and drapes should be removed quickly to prevent further damage from smoldering materials. Once the fire is extinguished, airway control must be quickly reestablished with a new ETT or tracheostomy.[46]

The powered microdebrider (Xomed, Jacksonville, FL, USA) has been proved to be a useful modality for the endoscopic management of an obstructing airway tumor. The instrument can be maneuvered through a rigid bronchoscope, tracheoscope, or laryngoscope. This device uses a suction cannula containing a variety of spinning blades, thus permitting simultaneous fragmentation of the tumor with removal of the debris. Recent case series have shown that 53% to 100% of patients treated with this modality have resulted in fully patent airway without evidence of residual tumor.[44,47]

Airway stents

Endoscopic airway stenting can be a good treatment option for patients who present with central airway occlusion secondary to extrinsic compression or tumor obstruction that has been partially debrided to allow accommodation of the stent. Stents are available in silicon-based varieties and self-expanding metallic stents, each with their own salient advantages and disadvantages. The silicon-based stent allows for easy repositioning and removal because of its low propensity for granulation tissue formation. Unfortunately, these stents have a higher rate of migration up to 17% and are susceptible to significant inspissated mucus, thus requiring frequent reinterventions.[48] Also, the silastic stents require rigid bronchoscopy for placement.

Contrastingly, the self-expanding metallic stents have adequate radial force to fill the tracheobronchial lumen, which decreases the chance of trapped secretions. These stents can be placed with flexible bronchoscopy under fluoroscopic guidance. However, because of their metal lattice, they become well ingrained into the tracheobronchial mucosa.[49] In addition, these stents promote the formation of significant granulation tissue, which may require repeat interventions for debridement. Silastic covered metallic stents are available, which may prevent the embedding of the stent into the airway wall. Nevertheless, the uncovered ends of the stent still allow significant tissue ingrowth. Tissue ingrowth rates of up to 33% have been reported, using the metallic self-expanding stents, and preclude its frequent use in benign stenoses.[50] Cohort studies examining the difference in outcomes between self-expanding metallic stents in malignant and benign disease showed a complication rate that was doubled in the benign population (21% vs 42%).[51]

Unfortunately, the airway stent itself can be the cause of an airway obstruction. An occluded or migrated stent can lead to hypoventilation, hypoxia, and loss of the airway. This clinical scenario requires prompt rigid or flexible bronchoscopy for diagnosis and treatment. Inspissated secretions can usually be cleaned with bronchoscopic irrigation and suctioning. Owing to their low propensity for ingrowth, silicone stents can often be removed and replaced easily if unable to debride. Significant ingrowth of tumor or granulation tissue often found with metallic stents requires adjunct recanalization and tissue destruction techniques, as discussed earlier referencing the article by Wood.[52]

Tissue destruction

Removal of a tumor causing an acute central airway obstruction and identifying the true airway lumen is the primary goal. In an emergent setting, this is best accomplished with rigid bronchoscopy and recanalization as described previously. Although not usually applicable to a crisis, techniques that induce tissue destruction are also occasionally used and should be available. Although a detailed description is beyond the scope of this article, these include

- Neodymium:yttrium-aluminum-garnet laser or CO_2 laser
- Argon plasma coagulation
- Standard electrocautery
- Photodynamic therapy
- Cryotherapy

Postoperative Management

After the definitive procedure has been completed, the airway should be thoroughly suctioned and hemostasis achieved. The patient can be ventilated with the rigid bronchoscope until awake and ready for extubation. However, conversion to an endotracheal tube or laryngeal mask airway is often better tolerated. It is important to keep all endoscopic equipment, along with necessary adjuncts, in the operating room and immediately attainable. In addition, the surgeon should not leave the room until confirmation from the anesthesiologist or successful extubation. Postoperative subglottic edema can be best managed with racemic epinephrine (0.2 mL of a 2% solution) or dexamethasone (4 mg intravenously every 6 hours). Improvement in symptoms occurs in 51% to 76% of patients after endoscopic intervention for central airway obstruction. Benign conditions tend to fair better postoperatively in terms of symptom reduction.[51]

SUMMARY

Successful airway stabilization in airway obstruction permits for temporization of life-threatening symptoms and planning for definitive surgical correction. Although quite stressful, the effective treatment of an acute central airway obstruction can be accomplished with a systematic approach using clear communication between teams and a comprehensive knowledge of available therapeutic modalities by the surgeon.

REFERENCES

1. Karzai W, Schwarzkopf K. Hypoxemia during one-lung ventilation: prediction, prevention, and treatment. Anesthesiology 2009;110(6):1402–11.
2. Durbin CG Jr, Rostow SK. More reliable oximetry reduces the frequency of arterial blood gas analyses and hastens oxygen weaning after cardiac surgery: a prospective, randomized trial of the clinical impact of a new technology. Crit Care Med 2002;30(8): 1735–40.
3. Chubra-Smith NM, Grant RP, Jenkins LC. Perioperative transcutaneous oxygen monitoring in thoracic anesthesia. Can Anaesth Soc J 1986;33(6):745–53.
4. Gelsomino S, Lorusso R, Livi U, et al. Assessment of a continuous blood gas monitoring system in animals during circulatory stress. BMC Anesthesiol 2011;11:1.
5. Mahal I, Davie SN, Grocott HP. Cerebral oximetry and thoracic surgery. Curr Opin Anaesthesiol 2014;27(1):21–7.
6. MacLeod BA, Heller MB, Gerard J, et al. Verification of endotracheal tube placement with colorimetric end-tidal CO2 detection. Ann Emerg Med 1991; 20(3):267–70.
7. Cox P, Tobias JD. Noninvasive monitoring of PaCO(2) during one-lung ventilation and minimal access surgery in adults: End-tidal versus transcutaneous techniques. J Minim Access Surg 2007; 3(1):8–13.
8. Björk VO, Carlens E. The prevention of spread during pulmonary resection by the use of a double-lumen catheter. J Thorac Surg 1950;20(1):151–7.
9. Campos JH. Which device should be considered the best for lung isolation: double-lumen endotracheal tube versus bronchial blockers. Curr Opin Anaesthesiol 2007;20(1):27–31.
10. Brodsky JD. Con: proper positioning of a double-lumen endotracheal tube can only be accomplished with the use of endoscopy. J Cardiothorac Anesth 1988;2:105–9.

11. Campos JH. Progress in lung separation. Thorac Surg Clin 2005;15:71–83.
12. Brodksy JD, Macario A, Mark JBD. Tracheal diameter predicts double-lumen tube size: a method for selecting left double-lumen tubes. Anesth Analg 1996;82:861–4.
13. Hannallah M, Benumof JL, Silverman PM, et al. Evaluation of an approach to choosing a left double-lumen endobronchial tube size based on chest computed tomographic scan measurements of the left mainstem bronchial diameter. J Cardiothorac Vasc Anesth 1997;11:168–71.
14. Eberle B, Weiler N, Vogel N, et al. Computed tomography-based tracheobronchial image reconstruction allows selection of the individually appropriate double-lumen tube size. J Cardiothorac Vasc Anesth 1999;13:532–7.
15. Brodsky JD, Benumof JL, Ehrenwerth J. Depth of placement of left double-lumen endobronchial tubes. Anesth Analg 1991;73:570–2.
16. Alliaume BA, Coddens J, Deloof T. Reliability of auscultation in positioning of double-lumen endobronchial tubes. Can J Anaesth 1992;39:687–90.
17. Sivalingam P, Tio R. Tension pneumothorax, pneumomediastinum, pneumoperitoneum, and subcutaneous emphysema in a 15-year-old Chinese girl after a double-lumen tube intubation and one-lung ventilation. J Cardiothorac Vasc Anesth 1999;13: 312–5.
18. Torrance R, Dawson A, Wohlgemut JM, et al. Sudden loss of ventilation through a double-lumen endotracheal tube requiring a surgical bronchotomy. Ann Thorac Surg 2013;96(2):687–8.
19. Vas L, Naregal F, Nobre S, et al. Anaesthetic management for a left pneumonectomy in a child with bronchopleural fistula. Paediatr Anaesth 2000;10: 210–4.
20. Kaur D, Anand S, Sharma P, et al. Early presentation of postintubation tracheoesophageal fistula: Perioperative anesthetic management. J Anaesthesiol Clin Pharmacol 2012;28:114–6.
21. Campos JH. An update on bronchial blockers during lung separation techniques in adults. Anesth Analg 2003;97:1266–74.
22. Asai T. Failure of the Univent bronchial blocker in sealing the bronchus [letter]. Anaesthesia 1999; 54:97.
23. Bauer C, Winter C, Hentz JG, et al. Bronchial blocker compared to double-lumen tube for one-lung ventilation during thoracoscopy. Acta Anaesthesiol Scandal 2001;45(2):250–4.
24. Campos JH, Kernstine KH. A comparison of a left-sided Broncho-Cath, with the torque control blocker Univent and the wire-guided blocker. Anesth Analg 2003;96:283–9.
25. Kim H, Kim HK, Choi YH, et al. Thoracoscopic bleb resection using two-lung ventilation anesthesia with low tidal volume for primary spontaneous pneumothorax. Ann Thorac Surg 2009;87:880–5.
26. Sancheti MS, Dewan BP, Pickens A, et al. Thoracoscopy without lung isolation utilizing single lumen endotracheal tube intubation and carbon dioxide insufflation. Ann Thorac Surg 2013;96(2):439–44.
27. Force SD, Pelaez A, Neujahr DC, et al. Technique of right single-lung transplantation for idiopathic pulmonary fibrosis using cross-field ventilation. J Thorac Cardiovasc Surg 2007;133(1):272–3.
28. Grillo HC. Urgent treatment of tracheal obstruction. In: Grillo HC, editor. Surgery of the trachea and bronchi. Hamilton (Ontario): BC Decker; 2004. p. 471–8.
29. Bolliger CT, Mathur PN. ERS/ATS statement of interventional pulmonology. Eur Respir J 2002;19: 356–73.
30. Cavaliere S, Venuta F, Foccoli P, et al. Endoscopic treatment of malignant airway obstructions in 2,008 patients. Chest 1996;110:1536–42.
31. Ernst A, Feller-Kopman D, Becker HD, et al. Central airway obstruction. Am J Respir Crit Care Med 2004; 160:1278–97.
32. Williamson JP, Phillips MJ, Hillman DR, et al. Managing obstruction of the central airways. Intern Med J 2010;40(6):399–410.
33. Alfille P. Anesthesia for tracheal surgery. In: Grillo HC, editor. Surgery of the trachea and bronchus. Hamilton (Ontario): BC Decker; 2004. p. 453–70.
34. Conacher ID. Anaesthesia and tracheobronchial stenting for central airway obstruction in adults. Br J Anaesth 2003;90(3):367–74.
35. Lang G, Ghanim B, Hötzenecker K, et al. Extracorporeal membrane oxygenation support for complex tracheo-bronchial procedures. Eur J Cardiothorac Surg 2015;47(2):250–6.
36. Wood DE. Management of malignant tracheobronchial obstruction. Surg Clin North Am 2002;82: 621–42.
37. Grillo HC, Mathisen DJ. Primary tracheal tumors: treatment and results. Ann Thorac Surg 1990;49: 69–77.
38. Chao YK, Liu YH, Hsieh WJ, et al. Controlling difficult airway by rigid bronchoscope – an old but effective method. Interact Cardiovasc Thorac Surg 2005;4: 175–9.
39. Ost DE, Ernst A, Grosu HB, et al. Therapeutic bronchoscopy for malignant central airway obstruction: success rates and impact on dyspnea and quality of life. Chest 2015;147(5):1282–98.
40. Venuta F, Rendina EA, De Giacomo T, et al. Operative endoscopy of the airway with the old-fashioned esophageal dilators. Ann Thorac Surg 2005;79(2):718–9.
41. Chang AC, Pickens A, Orringer MB. Awake tracheobronchial dilation without the use of rigid bronchoscopy. Ann Thorac Surg 2006;82(6):e43–5.

42. Mayse ML, Greenheck J, Friedman M, et al. Successful bronchoscopic balloon dilation of nonmalignant tracheobronchial obstruction without fluoroscopy. Chest 2004;126(2):634–7.
43. Shitrit D, Kuchuk M, Zismanov V, et al. Bronchoscopic balloon dilatation of tracheobronchial stenosis: long-term follow-up. Eur J Cardiothorac Surg 2010;38(2):198–202.
44. Casal RF, Iribarren J, Eapen G, et al. Safety and effectiveness of microdebrider bronchoscopy for the management of central airway obstruction. Respirology 2013;18(6):1011–5.
45. Roy S, Smith LP. What does it take to start an oropharyngeal fire? Oxygen requirements to start fires in the operating room. Int J Pediatr Otorhinolaryngol 2011;75(2):227–30.
46. DeMaria S Jr, Schwartz AD, Narine V, et al. Management of intraoperative airway fire. Simul Healthc 2011;6(6):360–3.
47. Lunn W, Garland R, Ashiku S, et al. Microdebrider bronchoscopy: a new tool for the interventional bronchoscopist. Ann Thorac Surg 2005;80(4):1485–8.
48. Martinez-Ballarin JI, Diaz-Jimenez JP, Castro MJ, et al. Silicone stents in the management of benign tracheobronchial stenoses. Tolerance and early results in 63 patients. Chest 1996;109(3):626–9.
49. Lund ME, Force S. Airway stenting for patients with benign airway disease and the Food and Drug Administration advisory: a call for restraint. Chest 2007;132(4):1107–8.
50. Saad CP, Murthy S, Krizmanich G, et al. Self-expandable metallic airway stents and flexible bronchoscopy: long-term outcomes analysis. Chest 2003;124(5):1993–9.
51. Chung FT, Chen HC, Chou CL, et al. An outcome analysis of self-expandable metallic stents in central airway obstruction: a cohort study. J Cardiothorac Surg 2011;6:46.
52. Wood DE. Airway Stenting. Chest Surg Clin N Am 2003;13:211–29.

Operative and Perioperative Pulmonary Emboli

Jordy C. Cox, MD, David M. Jablons, MD*

KEYWORDS

- Pulmonary emboli • Operative • Perioperative • Venous thromboembolism
- Pulmonary embolectomy

KEY POINTS

- Intraoperative and perioperative massive pulmonary embolism (PE) remains an unusual but well-established cause of death; improved outcomes rely on a high index of suspicion, prompt recognition, and aggressive intervention.
- Surgical embolectomy outcomes have improved drastically since inception of this technique at the turn of the previous century; the procedure should be used without hesitation during an intraoperative crisis in which PE has been determined to be the cause.
- For patients with echocardiographic findings suggestive of ventricular dysfunction but who remain normotensive, the question of whether they should undergo surgical embolectomy or thrombolysis remains unanswered.
- When a thromboembolic event is suspected intraoperatively, transesophageal echocardiography seems to be the most reliable adjunct to diagnosis.
- In the setting of hemodynamic instability and echocardiographic evidence of right-heart strain, emergent surgical embolectomy should be considered and initiation of anticoagulation should not be delayed. This point is especially relevant in cases such as neurosurgery whereby systemic thrombolysis is likely to have severe hemorrhagic complications that are not easily correctible.
- For institutions that lack cardiopulmonary bypass capabilities, on-table systemic thrombolysis is likely to be the best treatment option. Use of advanced mechanical circulatory support (veno-arterial extracorporeal membrane oxygenation) may provide a reliable temporizing adjunct while off-loading the right ventricle and improving gas exchange.

INTRODUCTION

A 17-year-old boy was admitted to a trauma center following a head-on collision. He had been returning home after watching a basketball game and wearing only a lap belt. The shear forces caused a disruption of his anterior abdominal wall, multiple intestinal avulsions, and a spine fracture with spinal cord injury and paraplegia. He was taken emergently to surgery. The postoperative course was unremarkable. On postoperative day 5, the decision was made to electively place a prophylactic inferior vena cava (IVC) filter. He was taken back to the operating room (OR) where a femoral approach was chosen. The initial scout venogram was concerning for a filling defect in the iliac vein, but repeat imaging was clear. As the deployment system was advanced into position, the anesthesiologist noted a precipitous decrease in end-tidal carbon dioxide (CO_2). This decrease was followed by cardiac arrest. Cardiopulmonary

The authors have nothing to disclose.

UCSF Department of Surgery, UCSF Helen Diller Comprehensive Cancer Center at Mt Zion, 1600 Divisadero, St San Francisco, CA 94115, USA
* Corresponding author.
E-mail address: David.Jablons@ucsfmedctr.org

Thorac Surg Clin 25 (2015) 289–299
http://dx.doi.org/10.1016/j.thorsurg.2015.04.010
1547-4127/15/$ – see front matter

thoracic.theclinics.com

resuscitation (CPR) was initiated but unsuccessful at restoring hemodynamics.

Massive intraoperative pulmonary embolism (PE) is a rare event but carries high morbidity and mortality. Diagnosis remains a challenge; therapeutic approaches lack established consensus, especially in the setting of ongoing unrelated surgery. PE has been described as the most common cause of preventable death in hospitalized patients. Despite advances in prophylaxis, diagnostic approaches, and therapeutic modalities, it remains an underrecognized and lethal entity. Estimates suggest that PE is responsible for between 150,000 and 200,000 deaths per year in the United States (a third of which take place in the perioperative period). Several series have reported mortality rates ranging from 15% to 30%, especially when associated with hemodynamic instability. Venous thromboembolism (VTE) prevention has become the number one in-hospital safety improvement goal. The incidence of VTE in the major general surgery patient population without prophylaxis approaches 25% and can be as high as 60% in major trauma and 90% in spinal cord injuries.

In fatal cases of PE, it is known that death occurs within 1 hour of the embolism in 60% of cases.

Only 50% of deaths are attributed to massive emboli. The rest are caused by smaller submassive or recurrent events. The outcome is related to the size of the thrombus burden, the underlying cardiopulmonary function, and the promptness of diagnosis and institution of treatment. PE followed by cardiac arrest carries a 70% mortality. The potential survivors warrant aggressive intervention. PE associated with hemodynamic instability carries a 30% mortality, whereas PE that fails to produce right ventricular (RV) dilatation and hemodynamic compromise carries only a 1% mortality. Therefore, the presence of shock has traditionally defined the threshold for thrombolysis.

For a PE to become evident intraoperatively, it must have hemodynamic significance. PE should be included in the differential diagnosis of perioperative hypoxemia, hypotension, and hemodynamic compromise and a high index of suspicion must be maintained in order to ensure prompt recognition and treatment. This recognition is particularly difficult when patients have hemodynamic fluctuations during induction. The incidence of perioperative PE has been increasing. This increase is likely multifactorial but correlates with the increased rate of detection from more prevalent computed tomography (CT) scanning for diagnosis (**Fig. 1**). In this article, the authors attempt to define the best approach based on the most up-to-date publications and guidelines.

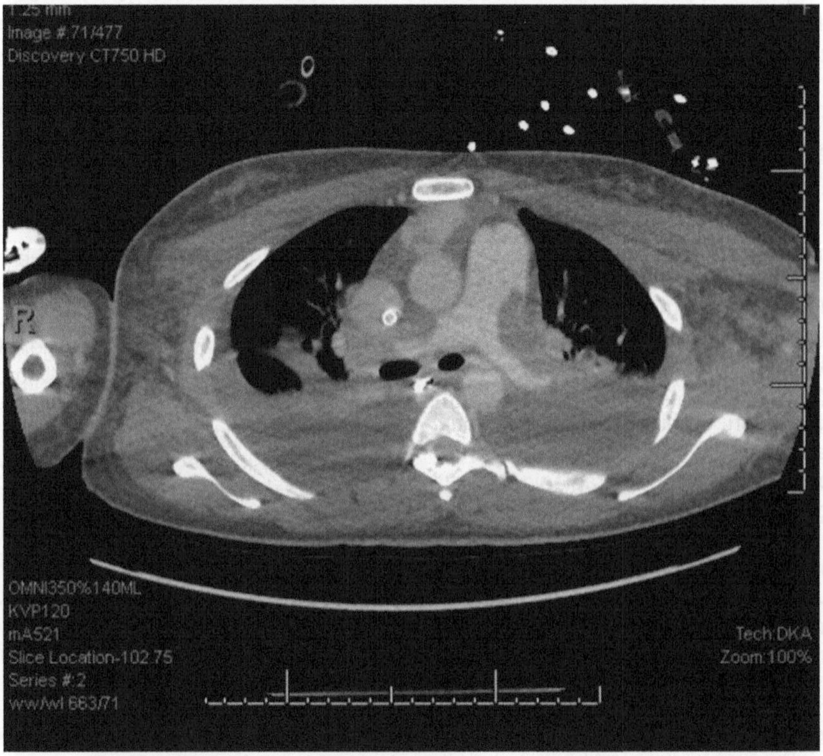

Fig. 1. Extensive emboli in right and left main pulmonary arteries.

RISK FACTORS

The Virchow triad of stasis (immobility, congestive heart failure), vessel injury (surgery or trauma), and hypercoagulability (malignancy, drug induced, oral contraceptives, hereditary) remain the basis for the development of VTE. Factors such as major orthopedic, abdominal, or pelvic surgery; trauma; prolonged immobilization; mechanical ventilation; use of neuromuscular blockers; presence of central venous catheters; and malignancy have all been associated with VTE formation. End-stage renal disease and other hypercoagulable states, such as activated protein C resistance, proteins C and S deficiencies, prothrombin mutations, and elevations in homocysteine, also predispose to VTE. Heparin-induced thrombocytopenia (HIT) results in an increased risk of VTE and arterial thrombosis.

PATHOPHYSIOLOGY

Most pulmonary emboli originate as VTEs in the deep veins of the lower extremities. Upper extremities and pelvic veins account for the rest. As the emboli lodges in the pulmonary artery (PA), platelet activation causes the release of vasoactive agents, such as histamine, activated complement, ADP, thromboxane, and serotonin, which increase pulmonary vascular resistance. The combination of mechanical outflow obstruction with an intense humoral response leads to substantial increases in RV afterload, which, in turn, lead to RV dilatation, ischemia, and dysfunction. The ensuing reduction in left ventricular (LV) filling and decreased coronary blood flow results in global cardiac dysfunction and hemodynamic collapse.

Because of its unique geometry, the RV is more sensitive to changes in pressure than to volume. Therefore, even small acute changes in pulmonary vascular resistance lead to dramatic changes in RV stroke volume (SV). In order to maintain this SV, there is a catecholamine-mediated increase in preload. Increased preload leads to RV dilatation, which shifts the septum and limits LV filling. As the LV SV decreases and overwhelms systemic compensatory vasoconstriction mechanisms, systemic hypoperfusion ensues.

PA obstruction leads to an increase in alveolar dead space and V/Q mismatch. This derangement is compounded by overperfusion of the nonobstructed portions of the pulmonary parenchyma and creates edema and alveolar hemorrhage. These changes persist long after the emboli themselves resolve. The presence of a patent foramen ovale (PFO) further worsens the condition as intracardiac shunting exacerbates hypoxemia and pulmonary vasoconstriction.

Despite adequate management, chronic thromboembolic pulmonary hypertension can result in approximately 5% of cases. These patients may eventually require pulmonary thromboendarterectomy and possibly transplantation should endarterectomy fail.

INTRAOPERATIVE DETECTION

Recognition of a PE in the perioperative period presents a substantial challenge, but early detection is paramount in reducing morbidity. Presenting symptoms cannot be seen in anesthetized patients; classic signs, such as tachycardia, hypoxia, and even shock, have multiple possible causes in the OR setting. Electrocardiogram changes include atrial arrhythmias, ST and T-wave abnormalities, and signs of right-heart strain, such as S1Q3T3, right-bundle-branch block, right axis deviation, or P pulmonale, as described by McGinn[1] in 1935. In patients who are breathing spontaneously, changes in the arterial blood gas analysis typically reflect hypoxemia, hypocapnia, and respiratory alkalosis. The most dramatic change, especially in the setting of a massive emboli, is a sudden and pronounced decrease in end-tidal CO_2.[2]

A normal D-dimer level, as demonstrated by an enzyme-linked immunosorbent assay (ELISA), has a sensitivity of 99% and safely excludes a PE. Its usefulness in the perioperative period is limited as fibrin is produced in conditions (such as trauma, malignancy, infection, and inflammation) that are typically part of the operative constellation.

Transesophageal echocardiography (TEE) with color-flow Doppler might be the only available accurate diagnostic tool that can be performed in the OR without interrupting the procedure. There are reports of endobronchial ultrasound (EBUS) accurately diagnosing a PE. Although this technique is uniquely suited to imaging the PA, it does, temporarily, partially obstruct the endotracheal tube and may worsen the hypoxia. This technology and the expertise to apply it are not always immediately available in a general OR. TEE and EBUS have the distinct advantage of being performed on the operating table as the main procedure is ongoing.

A recent study analyzed 146 cases of massive intraoperative PE and attempted to identify the best diagnostic tools: end-tidal CO_2, central venous pressures, echocardiography, and standard vital sign monitoring. Changes in end-tidal CO_2 were associated with the earliest detection and lowest mortality. Echocardiographic evidence of thrombus was noted in 87% of cases and indirect evidence of RV strain in 92%. RV dilatation, tricuspid regurgitation, and wall motion abnormalities were all associated with increased mortality. This retrospective review clearly supported the use of capnography as a screening tool and a low threshold for the use of intraoperative TEE as confirmatory test.[3]

The 2014 guidelines of the European Society of Cardiology's Task Force for the Diagnosis and Management of Acute Pulmonary Embolism regarding diagnosis of patients with suspected high-risk PE and shock establish that[4]

- Emergency CT angiogram (CTA) or bedside echography (depending on availability and clinical circumstances) is recommended for diagnostic purposes (class I recommendation, level of evidence C).
- In patients who are too unstable to undergo confirmatory CTA, bedside search for venous and/or PA thrombi with ultrasound and/or TEE may be considered to further support the diagnosis (class IIb recommendation, level of evidence C).
- Pulmonary angiography should be considered in unstable patients referred directly to the catheterization laboratory, in case once an acute coronary syndrome has been excluded, PE emerges as a possible diagnostic alternative (class IIb recommendation, level of evidence C).

A recent review of more than 3000 massive intraoperative thromboembolic events spanning 5 decades found an overall mortality of 41%. Thrombotic, neoplastic, and gaseous emboli were the most common causes. All types of surgery were involved and did not have a statistically significant bearing on outcomes. The use of a PA catheter was associated with improved mortality. Overall, therapeutic interventions resulted in better outcomes when compared with supportive care alone. Unfortunately, given the power of this study, the investigators were unable to find statistically significant differences in outcomes between the therapeutic options. However, mortality was greater in the systemic thrombolysis group than in any other. TEE was found to be a useful tool in the diagnosis and detection of postintervention improvements in RV wall motion abnormalities.[5]

INITIAL STABILIZATION AND MONITORING

Following a massive PE, hemodynamics are initially supported by an intense endogenous catecholamine release. Escalating oxygen requirements often call for intubation and mechanical ventilation. This intervention often precipitates cardiovascular collapse as the catecholamine surge is mitigated and drug-induced vasodilatation lowers preload and leads to subendocardial ischemia and cardiac decompensation. Moreover, positive pressure ventilation will decrease systemic venous return and increase pulmonary vascular resistance further jeopardizing RV function. The use of induction agents, such as etomidate or ketamine, is ideal as they cause less myocardial depression.

Although volume expansion with crystalloid solution is the initial treatment choice for any undifferentiated shock, in the PE-related crisis, fluid overload will significantly increase RV preload and systolic wall stress further worsening the ischemia. Therefore, consideration to early use of vasopressors and limiting resuscitation to 500 mL of crystalloid has been advocated, especially in the setting of compromised cardiac output and/or echocardiographic evidence of RV dysfunction.

Norepinephrine seems to be the agent of choice given how it increases mean arterial blood pressure (MABP) and enhances perfusion pressure gradients to the RV subendocardium. It also possesses a modest B1 inotropic effect that enhances RV contractility. Despite their attractive potential, inotropic agents, such as dobutamine, also cause peripheral vasodilatation through a B2 effect. Consideration should be given to the combined use of these two agents. It is also reasonable to consider the use of pulmonary vasodilators, such as inhaled prostacyclin or nitric oxide and parenteral sildenafil, given the vasoconstrictive neurohumoral response to PE. These agents may improve cardiac output and gas exchange.

The presence of shock or hemodynamic decompensation in patients with proven PE is an indication for thrombolysis or surgical embolectomy. This finding has been supported by multiple clinical trials. Bleeding complications from the thrombolytic therapy remain the major concern, especially in the intraoperative and immediate postoperative setting.

The different thrombolytic agents seem to have similar efficacy provided that equivalent doses are given over a similar period of time. Additionally, as shown by Verstraete and others[6], there seems to be no difference in efficacy between intrapulmonary thrombolytic therapy and peripheral intravenous (IV) thrombolytic therapy.

Echocardiography-based studies have shown that thrombi that are long, mobile, and hypoechoic are more susceptible to thrombolysis than those that are immobile and homogeneous/hyperechoic. When indirect signs of RV dysfunction are seen on echo, there is an association with increased mortality. Mortality in patients who fail to respond to thrombolytic therapy approaches 30%.

Assessing the efficacy of the intervention can also be challenging during the first few hours.

Monitoring of end-tidal CO_2 may be used as a barometer to define the need for additional interventions. Improvement in cardiac output, reduction of the degree of tricuspid regurgitation, and a decrease in central venous pressure are also indicators of improvement.

Biomarkers have also been used: B-type natriuretic peptide (BNP) as an indicator of RV stress and troponin I and T levels as indicators of myocardial ischemia can be monitored and their trend followed. In the absence of hemodynamic instability and elevation of these markers, the predicted outcome has been shown to be excellent. In contrast, elevations of BNP and troponin isoenzymes are associated with higher mortality. Their utility as discriminators for the initiation of thrombolytic therapy is growing.[7,8] For those that fail thrombolysis, there seems to be a significant survival benefit in undertaking surgical embolectomy. The incidence of recurrent PE is higher in patients requiring repeat thrombolysis and is also a significant cause of death. The use of IVC filters in this setting may significantly impact this.

The 2006 Cochrane review reported poor outcomes in those patients with greater than 70% of initial pulmonary vascular obstruction, hemodynamic instability at presentation, paradoxic septal motion on echo, older age, and residual vascular obstruction of greater than 30% after thrombolysis.

Surgical embolectomy should be considered for emboli presenting with shock and in when systemic thrombolysis is contraindicated. Ideally, the emboli are large and centrally located, and embolectomy is undertaken before cardiac arrest. This procedure typically requires localization with CT imaging and/or echocardiography. Whenever an intraoperative PE is suspected, TEE should be used.

VENOUS THROMBOEMBOLISM IN THORACIC SURGERY PATIENTS

The occurrence of a VTE in patients who have undergone thoracic and cardiac surgery is associated with significant morbidity and mortality. The incidence of VTE in post–coronary artery bypass graft surgery patients has been reported at around 20%. Less than 1% of these develop a PE. Mortality, however, can be as high as 20%. VTEs have been found in both the extremity that is the site of saphenous vein harvest and in the nonharvested extremity. Ultrasonography will reliably detect a proximal VTE in 50% of patients with a PE. A normal ultrasound of the leg veins does not rule out PE.

Recognition of VTE and PE is difficult in the post-thoracic surgery patient population. Cardinal symptoms of leg swelling and pain are common in an extremity that has undergone vein harvesting. Dyspnea, mild hypoxia, and chest pain are also common following thoracotomy or sternotomy. Atelectasis, pleural effusions, pain, fluid overload, atrial fibrillation, and cardiac dysfunction have shared presentations with and can easily mask an embolic event. Previously mentioned biomarkers (BNP and troponin) are also commonly abnormal following thoracic surgery.

A high index of suspicion is critical in the identification of patients at risk and those that have developed a thromboembolic complication. The main diagnostic tool is currently a multidetector CTA, with a reported sensitivity and specificity of 83% and 96%, respectively. This finding was initially validated by the PIOPED II (Prospective Investigation of Pulmonary Embolism Diagnosis) trial.[9]

PREVENTION

Based on the American College of Chest Physicians' 2012 evidence-based clinical practice guidelines on antithrombotic therapy and prevention of thrombosis, ninth edition, the following is recommended[10]:

For patients undergoing cardiac surgery, mechanical prophylaxis in the form of intermittent pneumatic compression for an uncomplicated postoperative course is used, with the addition of a pharmacologic prophylaxis (low-molecular-weight heparin [LMWH] or low-dose unfractionated heparin [UH]) for a prolonged course complicated by nonhemorrhagic events (grade 2C recommendations).

For patients undergoing thoracic surgery, use mechanical and pharmacologic prophylaxis in patients at moderate risk for VTE who are not at high risk for perioperative bleeding (grade 1B recommendations) and mechanical prophylaxis only in those cases at high risk for perioperative bleeding until such time as the bleeding risk diminishes (grade 2C recommendations).

TREATMENT

The American College of Chest Physicians' 2012 evidence-based clinical practice guidelines on antithrombotic therapy and prevention of thrombosis, ninth edition, recommends the following:

For the initial treatment of a VTE/PE, use LMWH or fondaparinux over IV or subcutaneous UH for at least 5 days and until the international normalized ratio (INR) is greater than 2.0 followed by 3 months of oral anticoagulation therapy with vitamin K antagonists and an INR target of 2.5 (range 2–3).

Twice-daily dosing of parenteral agents is preferred, and vitamin K antagonists should be started on the same day that parenteral anticoagulation is initiated (grade 1B recommendation).

The 2014 guidelines of the European Society of Cardiology's Task Force for the Diagnosis and Management of Acute Pulmonary Embolism indicate that once acute-phase parenteral anticoagulation has been initiated, acceptable alternatives to vitamin K antagonists include apixaban, dabigatran, and edoxaban. These agents should not be used in patients with severe renal impairment (creatinine clearance <30 mL/min). These recommendations are class I and supported by levels of evidence B.[4]

In pregnancy, a weight-adjusted dose of LMWH is the recommended therapy.

HEPARIN-INDUCED THROMBOCYTOPENIA

HIT is an immune-mediated disorder caused by the development of immunoglobulin G antibodies against heparin when bound to the platelet factor 4 (PF4) protein. This disorder results in platelet activation and subsequent thrombus formation.

In cardiac surgical patients, the incidence of HIT is estimated to be 5%. It is associated with the use of UH but also LMWH. Life-threatening adverse effects are secondary to the development of thrombosis anywhere in the arterial and venous circulation and include both hemorrhagic and thromboembolic complications. HIT should be suspected when the platelet count decreases by 50% or more from baseline, in the absence of other causes of thrombocytopenia, and is associated with the development of new thrombosis or the extension of preexisting thrombosis within 5 to 10 days of exposure to heparin.

Diagnosis relies on laboratory assays. The serotonin release assay is the gold standard diagnostic test. It uses platelets and serum from patients and monitors for serotonin release, as a marker of platelet activation when combined with heparin. Although this test has a 95% sensitivity and specificity, it is slow and costly and used, therefore, for confirmation. The detection of antibodies against heparin-PF4 complexes is an antigenic ELISA test that is highly sensitive but less specific and is used as screening.

Management of patients with HIT is focused on the reduction of thrombus formation and a decrease in platelet activation. All forms of heparin must be stopped; given the strong predisposition to repeated thrombotic episodes, anticoagulation must be initiated with either direct thrombin inhibitors (argatroban, lepirudin, or bivalirudin) or factor Xa inhibitors (danaparoid, fondaparinux, dabigatran, or rivaroxaban). Platelet transfusion is discouraged as it may lead to worse thrombotic complications. All these agents carry a substantial risk of bleeding, potential anaphylaxis, and variable effectiveness given dependence on renal or hepatic metabolism.

THERAPEUTIC OPTIONS FOR THE TREATMENT OF ACUTE PULMONARY EMBOLISM

When faced with a perioperative PE, several options for treatment exist.

Anticoagulation

Anticoagulation is indicated for normotensive patients with normal RV function.

Systemic Thrombolysis

Systemic thrombolysis is indicated in patients who are normotensive but with evidence of RV dysfunction or in those cases of hemodynamic compromise.

Agents with proven effectiveness include streptokinase (SK), urokinase (UK), and recombinant tissue plasminogen activator (rtPA). They all seem to be similarly effective. The hemodynamic effects are particularly significant during the first few days, and the best outcomes are observed when infusion is begun within 48 hours of the onset of symptoms. The infusion regimen should be abbreviated (administration over 2 hours), and UH infusions should be stopped during administration of SK and UK but may be continued during rtPA.[4]

The effectiveness of this approach was set in the classic UPET (The Urokinase-Streptokinase Pulmonary Embolism) trial published in 1974.[11]

The 2008 guidelines of the European Society of Cardiology's Task Force for the Diagnosis and Management of Acute Pulmonary Embolism indicate the absolute contraindications to systemic thrombolytic therapy to be hemorrhagic stroke or stroke of unknown origin at the time of PE, ischemic stroke within 6 months, central nervous system (CNS) neoplasms, major trauma or surgery within the preceding 3 weeks, gastrointestinal bleeding within the last month, and known active bleeding.

Relative contraindications are transient ischemic stroke within the last 6 months, oral anticoagulant therapy, advanced hepatic disease, infective endocarditis, retinal hemorrhage, pregnancy or less than 1 week postpartum, active peptic ulcer, recent resuscitation, refractory hypertension (>180 mm Hg), and severe thrombocytopenia.[12]

The role of systemic thrombolytic therapy in the post–cardiac surgery patient population is limited given the consequences of bleeding complications. However, traditional contraindications to anticoagulation are considered relative in the setting of a PE with hemodynamic collapse and a patient in extremis who is proving refractory to other therapeutic interventions. Complications from this approach include an increased risk of serious bleeding. The overall incidence of major hemorrhage is reportedly around 12%; particularly, there is a 1% to 3% incidence of intracranial hemorrhage that can be fatal in up to 50% of cases.[13,14]

Catheter Embolectomy or Catheter-Directed Thrombolysis

Catheter embolectomy or catheter-directed thrombolysis is considered in cases of failure of systemic thrombolysis, contraindications to thrombolytic therapy, and when surgical embolectomy is unavailable or not feasible.

Several variants of this technology are available: rheolytic embolectomy uses pressurized saline; rotational embolectomy fragments the thrombi using a mechanical device; and suction embolectomy uses negative pressure to aspirate the clot. Most cause thrombus fragmentation and achieve varying degrees of completeness of thrombus removal, ranging from 40% to 100%. Delivery sheaths vary in size from 6 to 11 French. Those devices that require cut down of the jugular vein for delivery (such as the Rheolytic system) have an increased risk of local vascular complications and hemorrhage.[15]

Pulmonary Embolectomy

Pulmonary embolectomy is indicated in critical patients in which there has been a failure of systemic thrombolysis and/or catheter embolectomy or in whom there is insufficient time for effective thrombolytic therapy. Recent data have shown that surgical embolectomy has superior outcomes when compared with repeat thrombolysis.[16] Surgical embolectomy should also be considered in the setting of intracardiac thrombi or systemic embolic complications from an emboli in transit through a PFO or other septal defects.

The 2014 guidelines of the European Society of Cardiology's Task Force for the Diagnosis and Management of Acute Pulmonary Embolism regarding treatment of patients with suspected high-risk PE and shock/hypotension state[4]

- IV anticoagulation with UH must be initiated without delay (class I recommendation, level of evidence C).
- Thrombolytic therapy is recommended (class I recommendation, level of evidence B).
- Surgical embolectomy is recommended for patients in whom thrombolysis is contraindicated or has failed (class I recommendation, level of evidence C).
- Percutaneous catheter-directed treatment should be considered as an alternative to surgical embolectomy for patients in whom full-dose systemic thrombolysis is contraindicated or has failed (class IIa recommendation, level of evidence C).

PULMONARY EMBOLECTOMY

On the afternoon of October 3, 1930, Dr Edward Churchill was called to the bedside of a woman who had been recovering from a cholecystectomy. She was complaining of chest pain and dyspnea and was deteriorating rapidly. A massive PE was suspected. A young trainee monitored her until the following morning when she further decompensated. Dr Churchill opened the chest and performed a Trendelenburg embolectomy in less than 10 minutes, but the patient never regained consciousness. The trainee that had been assigned to the bedside watch was Dr John Heysham Gibbon, Jr and he credits this episode as the catalyst that lead him to the development of the heart-lung machine and the first successful operation under cardiopulmonary bypass nearly 3 decades later.[17]

Early descriptions of the surgical removal of pulmonary emboli are credited to Dr Friedrich Trendelenburg, surgeon-in-chief at the University of Leipzig in the early 1900s. His student, Martin Kirschner, is considered to have performed the first successful procedure on March 18, 1924. More recent successes without the use of cardiopulmonary bypass date back to the early 1960s when hypothermia and venous inflow occlusion provided modest results. The first successful pulmonary embolectomy with extracorporeal circulation is credited to EH Sharp in 1962.[18]

Technological improvements, especially those related to cardiopulmonary bypass, have drastically impacted the outcomes of the procedure, with recent reported mortality in the 5% range. Given this decline, it has recently been suggested that indications for surgical embolectomy be expanded and not reserved exclusively for those patients who have failed thrombolysis.

Emboli that are most amenable to surgical extraction are limited to the proximal main PAs. Identification with spiral CT is ideal before proceeding with surgery. Spiral CT has been validated and has replaced pulmonary angiography as the primary imaging modality for diagnosis. It is also a useful adjunct in the detection of intracardiac and extracardiac causes of thromboembolism.

Echocardiography is a useful diagnostic tool for visualizing centrally located emboli. It is also useful in the detection of RV dysfunction and can identify other intracardiac, such as septal defects and intracardiac thrombi. It is also a helpful adjunct in the monitoring of the RV and its response to treatment. Indirect signs of concern are paradoxic septal motion, tricuspid valve regurgitation (with a jet velocity >2.8 m/s), and IVC congestion. Its primary limitation resides in detecting emboli located in the main left PA. Several investigators advocate that TEE has limited sensitivity and that failure to demonstrate a thrombus does not exclude the need for intervention.[19] The echocardiographic criterion of RV enlargement is defined as a diameter of 90% or greater of the size of the LV.

INDICATIONS FOR SURGICAL EMBOLECTOMY

Most patients with acute pulmonary emboli do not require surgical intervention. Traditionally, this approach has been reserved for those with a massive PE that has been confirmed by imaging, who have hemodynamic instability despite anticoagulation and failure (or absolute contraindication to) systemic thrombolytic therapy (or insufficient time for it to be effective).

The presence of intracardiac, such as a free-floating thrombus or a trapped thrombi within a PFO/atrial septal defect, are also indications for surgical intervention.

A definitive diagnosis is ideal before intervention. If preoperative imaging is not an option given the urgency or because of an intraoperative crisis, an emergent TEE with color-flow Doppler should be used to help confirm the presence of an embolism. Typically, these patients are already in a profound state of hemodynamic compromise; additional delays for confirmatory studies can lead to poor outcomes. In cases in which the luxury of confirmatory testing is not afforded, the decision to proceed with a rescue embolectomy may be feasible and should be entertained.

SURGICAL TECHNIQUE

Approach is via a median sternotomy. The pericardium is entered; after systemic heparinization, aortic and bicaval cannulation is used. The use of cardioplegic or fibrillatory arrest and aortic cross-clamping versus beating heart technique is left at the surgeon's discretion. Normothermia is usually maintained given the short period of bypass.

The main PA trunk is exposed, and a longitudinal arteriotomy is performed 2 cm distal to the pulmonic valve with extension onto the proximal left PA. The thrombi are extracted under direct vision. Right-angled Dejardin gallstone forceps are helpful. Gentle irrigation and, occasionally, a Fogarty balloon embolectomy catheter are used to access the most peripheral clots. Gentle compression of the lung parenchyma can also assist in dislodging smaller distal thrombi. Additionally, a longitudinal right PA incision between the superior vena cava and the aorta can be used to improve access and visualization. A pediatric bronchoscope or a choledocoscope can be used for direct visualization of the arterial tree and confirmation that all major branches are free of thrombus. Removal of thrombi to the segmental level is usually achieved.

The PA is a delicate structure. Gentle manipulation is mandatory to avoid injury that might prove extremely challenging (if not impossible) to repair. If indicated, removal of RA or RV thrombus and closure of PFO is accomplished also. The arteriotomy is closed with a running suture, and patients are weaned from cardiopulmonary bypass (**Fig. 2**).

The placement of an IVC filter to decrease the incidence of recurrent emboli is often done concomitantly but no consensus exists over its use. The 2014 guidelines of the European Society of Cardiology's Task Force for the Diagnosis and Management of Acute Pulmonary Embolism regarding the use of IVC filters following a PE state that[4]

- IVC filters should be considered in patients with acute PE and absolute contraindications to anticoagulation (class IIa recommendation, level of evidence C).
- IVC filters should be considered in cases of recurrent PE despite therapeutic levels of anticoagulation (class IIa recommendation, level of evidence C).

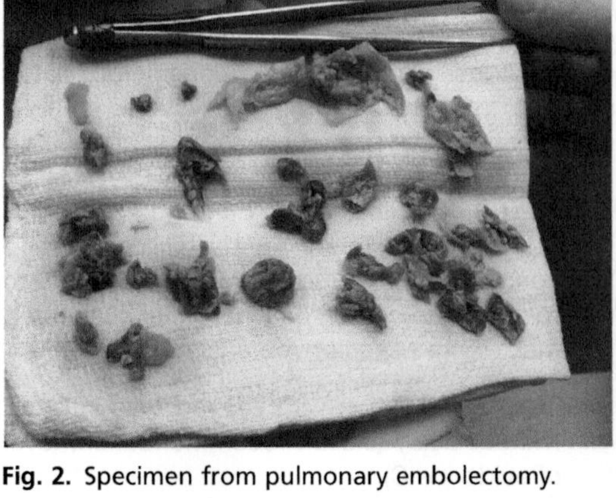

Fig. 2. Specimen from pulmonary embolectomy.

- Routine use of IVC filters in patients with PE is not recommended (class III recommendation, level of evidence A).

Injury to the distal branches of the PA during embolectomy can lead to significant bronchoalveolar hemorrhage and manifest as significant hemoptysis and is particularly challenging in the setting of full heparinization. This can be worsened by reperfusion injury following resumption of pulmonary blood flow. Temporary isolation of the injured arterial branch with a ballooned catheter and increased PEEP can also assist with hemostasis. Isolation with a double lumen ETT and selective lung ventilation may be necessary in the more extreme cases. Bronchoscopy is useful to identify and located the bleeding. Resection of the involved parenchymal segment may be indicated.

Preoperative thrombolysis does increase intraoperative bleeding during the thrombectomy, but it does not constitute a contraindication to surgery.

Inability to wean from cardiopulmonary bypass because of primary RV dysfunction, persistent severe pulmonary hypertension (especially in the setting of acute-on-chronic pulmonary emboli), or severe hypoxia might require the use of mechanical circulatory support/extracorporeal membrane oxygenation (ECMO) as a bridge to recovery. The presence of an IVC filter limits venous cannula placement.

The use of mechanical circulatory support systems as an initial approach to rapidly deteriorating patients in order to sustain hemodynamics and provide right heart support has yet to be validated but offers an attractive temporizing measure that can be performed at bedside in the intensive care setting or intraoperatively and potentially allow transport of patients to tertiary care centers where definitive treatment can be achieved. Several recent reports from Japan have described the use of preoperative percutaneous venoarterial cardiopulmonary support with an overall mortality rate of only 12% in a cohort of high-risk patients that included those who had a cardiac arrest and had undergone CPR.[20,21] Venovenous circuits should not be used as they overload the RV.

POSTOPERATIVE ANTICOAGULATION

Current recommendations are to initiate systemic heparinization 6 hours after surgery as long as hemostasis seems adequate. Three months of oral anticoagulants are typically indicated except for episodes of recurrent emboli or those associated with noncorrectible causes, such as a malignancy, in which case anticoagulation should be lifelong.

PULMONARY EMBOLISM IN PREGNANCY

Acute PE is a known cause of death during pregnancy and may account for up to 20% of maternal deaths in the United States. As the body of literature supporting aggressive therapeutic modalities grows, some investigators have used this approach with success in acutely decompensated pregnant patients.[22]

The prevalence of PE during pregnancy is substantially higher than that of the general population. This prevalence is not only caused by the hypercoagulable state but also by mechanical compression of the IVC by the gravid uterus. Prompt diagnosis is crucial. Imaging tests can be performed safely, and radiation exposure levels are acceptable for the fetus.[4]

Systemic thrombolysis is relatively contraindicated. Consideration must be given to emergent delivery, especially if the fetus is of viable gestational age; but reports of successful term delivery exist. Heparin anticoagulation remains the initial treatment of choice; but catheter-directed thrombolysis, transcatheter thrombectomy, and surgical thrombectomy have all been used with good outcomes.

OTHER EMBOLIC SYNDROMES

PE can result from other materials. Fat, air, amniotic fluid, and silicone have been described. These pulmonary emboli can present acutely in the intraoperative and postoperative period and represent additional diagnostic and therapeutic challenges.

Gas emboli are typically iatrogenic in origin: insertion of central venous catheters, neurosurgical procedures, and inadequate deairing during cardiac surgery procedures are some of the more common causes. The clinical presentation can mimic that of standard PE, and a decrease in end-tidal CO_2 during surgery can alert a developing event. CO_2 emboli can occur during laparoscopic procedures. If suspected, insufflation should be stopped immediately. Several therapeutic modalities have been proposed. Positioning patients in the Trendelenburg position or in left lateral decubiti relies on trapping of the air in the RV. Aggressive resuscitation and CPR should be initiated promptly, and aggressive volume resuscitation has been proposed to increase right atrial pressures. Aspiration of air directly from right-sided cardiac chambers has also been done. There is no current established consensus regarding the management in these cases. Hyperbaric oxygen therapy has some use in the treatment of arterial cerebral air embolism but not for PE.

Fat embolism is most commonly seen in traumatic scenarios with long bone and pelvic fractures and at the time of surgical repair. The globules typically originate from exposed marrow or damaged adipose tissue. In addition to the mechanical effect of the globules, there seems to be a substantial activation of toxic mediator pathways, such as free-fatty acids and C-reactive protein, that may contribute to the constellation of symptoms that constitute fat emboli syndrome and lead to myocardial depression. The clinical scenario typically includes fever, dyspnea, hypoxemia, diffuse alveolar infiltrates, tachycardia, a petechial rash (anterior thorax, neck, and axillae), and CNS changes, such as seizures and alterations in the level of consciousness. These symptoms usually become manifest 1 to 3 days after the initial injury. Early immobilization of fractures reduces the incidence. Pulmonary changes can overlap acute lung injury/acute respiratory distress syndrome, and the diagnosis is usually one of exclusion and based on clinical findings. Treatment is mostly supportive, although the use of steroids and aspirin has been advocated to mitigate the proinflammatory pathways. Cerebral edema should be treated aggressively, and intracranial pressure monitoring is recommended. Hypovolemia should be avoided.

Amniotic fluid embolism is a potentially life-threatening event that occurs in the peripartum period. Although initially it was thought that mechanical embolization of amniotic fluid was responsible, more recent data suggest the syndrome results from activation of biochemical mediators in a fashion similar to fat emboli syndrome. It carries a high mortality rate from acute pulmonary hypertension secondary to vasospasm, myocardial depression, and disseminated intravascular coagulation and its associated complications. Symptoms commonly manifest during labor or in the immediate postpartum period. The classic presentation is that of dyspnea, hypoxia, hypotension, and eventually hemodynamic collapse and coagulopathy. CNS symptoms are also common. Diagnosis is one of exclusion, and treatment is mostly supportive.

Silicone embolism manifests clinically in a similar fashion to fat emboli syndrome. It usually occurs after silicone is injected in the setting of cosmetic surgical procedures. Hypoxia, fever, a petechial rash, and CNS alterations are common. Treatment in this event is supportive.

SUMMARY

Intraoperative and perioperative massive pulmonary emboli remain an unusual but well-established cause of death. Improved outcomes rely on a high index of suspicion, prompt recognition, and aggressive intervention.

Surgical embolectomy outcomes have improved drastically since its inception as a technique at the turn of the previous century and should be used without hesitation during an intraoperative crisis in which PE has been determined to be the cause. There is an emerging trend toward a more aggressive approach.

For those patients with echocardiographic findings suggestive of ventricular dysfunction but who remain normotensive, the question of whether they should undergo surgical embolectomy or thrombolysis remains unanswered.[23,24] When a thromboembolic event is suspected intraoperatively, a TEE seems to be the most reliable adjunct to diagnosis.

In the setting of hemodynamic instability and echocardiographic evidence of right-heart strain, emergent surgical embolectomy should be considered, and initiation of anticoagulation should not be delayed. This point is especially relevant in cases such as neurosurgery whereby systemic thrombolysis is likely to have severe hemorrhagic complications that are not easily correctible. For institutions that lack cardiopulmonary bypass capabilities, on-table systemic thrombolysis is likely to be the best treatment option. Use of advanced mechanical circulatory support (venoarterial ECMO) may provide a reliable temporizing adjunct while off-loading the right ventricle and improving gas exchange.

REFERENCES

1. McGinn S. Acute cor pulmonale resulting from pulmonary embolism. JAMA 1935;104:1473–80.
2. Desciak M, Martin D. Perioperative pulmonary embolism: diagnosis and anesthetic management. J Clin Anesth 2011;23:153–65.
3. Visnjevac O, Pourafkari L, Nader N. Role of perioperative monitoring in diagnosis of massive intraoperative cardiopulmonary embolism. J Cardiovasc Thorac Res 2014;6(3):141–5.
4. Konstantinides SV, Torbicki A, Agnelli G, et al, Task Force for the Diagnosis and Management of Acute Pulmonary Embolism of the European Society of Cardiology (ESC). 2014 ESC guidelines on the diagnosis and management of acute pulmonary embolism. Eur Heart J 2014;35(43):3033–69, 3069a–k.
5. Visnjevac O, Lee K, Bulatovic R, et al. Outcomes-based systematic review for management of massive intra-cardiac or pulmonary thrombotic emboli during surgery. Heart Lung Vessel 2014; 6(1):24–32.

6. Verstraete M, Miller A, Bounameaux H, et al. Intravenous and intrapulmonary recombinant tissue-type plasminogen activator in the treatment of acute massive pulmonary embolism. Circulation 1988; 77(2):353–60.
7. Cavallazzi R, Nair A, Vasu T, et al. Natriuretic peptides in acute pulmonary embolism: a systematic review. Intensive Care Med 2008;34:2147.
8. Becattini C, Vedovati M, Agnelli G. Prognostic value of troponins in acute pulmonary embolism: a meta-analysis. Circulation 2007;116:427.
9. Stein P, Fowler SE, Goodman LR, et al. Multidetector computed tomography for acute pulmonary embolism. N Engl J Med 2006;354(22):2317–27.
10. Holbrook A, Schulman S, Witt DM, et al. Evidence-based management of anticoagulant therapy: antithrombotic therapy and prevention of thrombosis, 9th ed: American College of Chest Physicians evidence based practice guidelines. Chest 2012;141(2 Suppl):e152S–84S.
11. Bell W, Simon T, Stengle J, et al. The Urokinase-Streptokinase pulmonary embolism trial (UPET). Circulation 1974;50:1070–1.
12. Torbicki A, Perrier A, Konstantinides S, et al, ESC Committee for Practice Guidelines (CPG). 2008 guidelines on the diagnosis and management of acute pulmonary embolism: the task force for the diagnosis and management of acute pulmonary of acute pulmonary embolism of the European Society of Cardiology. Eur Heart J 2008;29(18):2276–315.
13. Kanter D, Mikkola K, Patel S, et al. Thrombolytic therapy for pulmonary embolism. Frequency of intracranial hemorrhage and associated risk factors. Chest 1997;111(5):1241–5.
14. Levine M, Goldhaber S, Gore J, et al. Hemorrhagic complications of thrombolytic therapy in the treatment of myocardial infarction and venous thromboembolism. Chest 1995;108(4 Suppl):291S–301S.
15. Kucher N, Goldhaber S. Management of massive pulmonary embolism. Circulation 2005;112:e28–32.
16. Meneveau N, Seronde M, Blonde M, et al. Management of unsuccessful thrombolysis in acute massive pulmonary embolism. Chest 2006;129:1043.
17. Fou A. John H Gibbon. The first 20 years of the heart-lung machine. Tex Heart Inst J 1997;24(1):1–8.
18. Clarke D. Pulmonary embolectomy using normothermic venous inflow occlusion. Thorax 1968; 23:131.
19. Rosenberger P, Shernan S, Body S, et al. Utility of intraoperative transesophageal echocardiography for diagnosis of pulmonary embolism. Anesth Analg 2004;99:12–6.
20. Fukuda I, Taniguchi S, Fukui K, et al. Improved outcome of surgical pulmonary embolectomy by aggressive intervention for critically ill patients. Ann Thorac Surg 2011;91:728–33.
21. Takahashi H, Okada K, Matsumori M, et al. Aggressive surgical treatment of acute pulmonary embolism with circulatory collapse. Ann Thorac Surg 2012;94:785–91.
22. Saeed G, Moller M, Neuzner J, et al. Emergent surgical pulmonary embolectomy in a pregnant woman. Tex Heart Inst J 2014;41(2):188–94.
23. Worku B, Gulkarov I, Girardi L, et al. Pulmonary embolectomy in the treatment of submassive and massive pulmonary embolism. Cardiology 2014; 129:106–10.
24. Leacche M, Unic D, Goldhaber S, et al. Modern surgical treatment of massive pulmonary embolism: results in 47 consecutive patients after rapid diagnosis and aggressive surgical approach. J Thorac Cardiovasc Surg 2005;129:1018–23.

FURTHER READINGS

Nawas Z, Leeper K. Venous thromboembolism in the cardiac surgical patient. Chapter 282. In: Franco K, Thourani V, editors. Cardiothoracic surgery review. Philadelphia: Lippincott Williams & Wilkins; 2012. p. 1254–8.

Wood K, Joffe A. Pulmonary embolism. Chapter 142. In: Gabrielli A, Layon AJ, Yu M, editors. Critical care-Civetta, Taylor & Kirby. 4th edition. Philadelphia: Lippincott Williams & Wilkins; 2009. p. 2143–58.

Wood K. Major pulmonary embolism. Crit Care Clin 2011;27:885–906.

Acute Intraoperative Pulmonary Aspiration

Katie S. Nason, MD, MPH

KEYWORDS

• Anesthesia • Intratracheal • Intraoperative complications • Prevention and control • Pneumonia • Aspiration • Respiratory aspiration of gastric contents

KEY POINTS

- Thoracic surgery patients are at increased risk (threefold) for intraoperative aspiration compared with other surgical specialties.
- Aspiration pneumonitis is the most common sequela of significant intraoperative aspiration, followed by aspiration pneumonia.
- The severity of pulmonary parenchymal injury is modified by the degree of acidity, the volume of the aspirate, and the presence or absence of particulate matter in the aspirated fluid.
- Predisposing conditions include gastrointestinal obstruction, need for emergency surgery, previous esophageal surgery, esophageal cancer, hiatal hernia, impaired coordination of swallowing or respiration, and obesity.
- Preoperative assessment, appropriate fasting, and use of rapid-sequence induction, antisecretory medications, and rapid recognition/response to gastric regurgitation are critical to prevention and management.

INTRODUCTION

Although anesthesia is generally safe, respiratory complications such as anesthesia-related aspiration can be fatal.[1,2] Occurring as often as 1 in every 2000 to 3000 operations requiring anesthesia,[3] almost half of all patients who aspirate during surgery develop a related lung injury, such as pneumonitis or aspiration pneumonia.[4] This issue is of particular relevance to thoracic surgeons; Sakai and colleagues[5] retrospectively compared characteristics of patients with and without anesthetic-related pulmonary aspiration and found that aspiration occurred 3 times more often in thoracic surgical procedures than in any other specialty. As such, understanding the potential impact of anesthesia-related aspiration on perioperative outcomes, factors that contribute to an increased risk of this complication, and strategies for preventing the occurrence of or minimizing the sequela from an anesthesia-related aspiration are imperatives for the thoracic surgeon.

PULMONARY ASPIRATION: DEFINITION, CONSEQUENCES, AND RISK FACTORS

Definition and Consequences

Defined as the entry of liquid or solid material into the trachea and lungs, anesthesia-related aspiration occurs when patients without sufficient laryngeal protective reflexes passively or actively regurgitate gastric contents. Pulmonary syndromes of differing severity result, ranging from mild symptoms, such as hypoxia, to complete

Disclosure for Financial Support: Dr K.S. Nason is supported by the National Cancer Institute of the National Institutes of Health under award number 5K07CA151613. The content is solely the responsibility of the authors and does not necessarily represent the official views of the National Institutes of Health.
Division of Thoracic and Foregut Surgery, Department of Cardiothoracic Surgery, University of Pittsburgh, 5200 Centre Avenue, Suite 715, Shadyside Medical Building, Pittsburgh, PA 15232, USA
E-mail address: nasonks@upmc.edu

Thorac Surg Clin 25 (2015) 301–307
http://dx.doi.org/10.1016/j.thorsurg.2015.04.011
1547-4127/15/$ – see front matter

respiratory failure and acute respiratory distress syndrome (ARDS), and even cardiopulmonary collapse and death. The types of pulmonary syndromes include acid-associated pneumonitis, particle-associated aspiration (eg, airway obstruction), or bacterial infection, with subsequent development of lung abscess, exogenous lipoid pneumonia, chronic interstitial fibrosis, and *Mycobacterium fortuitum* pneumonia.[6] Which of these syndromes develops depends on the composition and volume of the aspirate.

The most common lung injury is aspiration pneumonitis. Initially described by Mendelson in 1946, aspiration pneumonitis is damage to the lung parenchyma resulting from inhalation of sterile, acid (or bile) gastric contents. The severity of pulmonary parenchymal injury is modified by the degree of acidity, the volume of the aspirate, and the presence or absence of particulate matter in the aspirated fluid. Low-volume aspirate with a very low pH can rapidly lead to fatal pneumonitis, whereas higher volumes of aspirate that are buffered (ie, higher pH) can be better tolerated. As little as 50 mL of regurgitated gastric contents can be considered a "severe" aspiration.[7] When the aspirate is not sterile or when particulate matter are present in the aspirate, mechanical airway obstruction and infectious complications can develop, with the most common pathogens being *Staphylococcus aureus*, *Pseudomonas aeruginosa*, *Enterobacter* species, anaerobes, *Klebsiella* species, and *Escherichia coli*.[8]

Risk Factors

There are a number of patient-related and procedure-related characteristics that place some patients at higher risk for an anesthesia-related aspiration event.

Risk factors: medications

In and of itself, anesthesia places patients at risk for aspiration. This risk results from the effects of medications on the lower esophageal sphincter, level of consciousness, and loss of protective reflexes.

There are a number of medications that are routinely used during anesthesia that are known to decrease lower esophageal sphincter tone.[9] These include the following:

- Propofol
- Volatile anesthetic agents
- β-agonists
- Opioids
- Atropine
- Thiopental
- Tricyclics
- Glycopyrrolate

In addition to effects on lower esophageal sphincter pressures, these medications by design induce a progressive loss of consciousness with subsequent decline and then loss of protective reflexes.[10] This risk is even greater when topical anesthesia to the larynx is used, because the cough reflex is compromised.[11]

Risk factors: predisposing conditions

It is important to note, however, that most patients undergoing anesthesia do not suffer from an aspiration event; predisposing conditions must also exist that, in combination with progressive loss of consciousness and diminished protective reflexes, create a favorable environment for aspiration. These predisposing conditions include[12] the following:

- Gastrointestinal obstruction
- Need for emergency surgery
- Previous esophageal surgery
- Esophageal cancer
- Hiatal hernia
- Lack of coordination of swallowing or respiration
- Obesity

Consistent with the upper gastrointestinal stasis and/or obstruction associated with most of these conditions, passive regurgitation with induction of general anesthesia is far more common than active vomiting.[13]

Risk factors: provider expertise

At least one study found that provider factors, such as improper decision-making, lack of experience, and lack of knowledge, were responsible for most intraoperative aspiration events.[14] Provider expertise also is implicated in failure of preventive measures, such as the use of cricoid pressure during rapid-sequence induction[15] (RSI) (see later in this article) and wide variation in the execution of these approaches to anesthesia induction in the high-risk patient. In the retrospective review of anesthesia-related aspirations by Sakai and colleagues,[5] 10 of the 14 cases were attributed to improper anesthesia technique. In their critical review of anesthetic management, they found that cricoid pressure was not applied at the time of induction in 4 cases, and provider inexperience contributed to aspiration in a high-risk patient in another patient. Kluger and Short[13] reported similar concerns regarding provider-specific factors in their review of 133 cases drawn from the New Zealand Anesthetic Incident Monitoring Study database. As with other studies, passive regurgitation was 3 times more common than active vomiting and most cases had at least one predisposing risk factor for regurgitation. Despite this, only 14% of the patients who aspirated had any antiaspiration prophylaxis (defined in the study as cricoid pressure, acid-suppression therapy, and prokinetic agents) used before and during induction. Factors contributing to the aspiration event were taken directly from the reports submitted to the database and included error in judgment (n = 43; including inadequate anesthesia), fault of technique (n = 35), inadequate patient preparation (n = 25), communication problem (n = 14), inadequate assistance (n = 14), and provider inexperience (n = 13).[13]

PREVENTION

Preoperative Risk Assessment

The key to minimizing the impact of acute intraoperative aspiration is to prevent it from happening. A thorough knowledge of the patient and their predisposing conditions, including a physical examination and review of current symptoms, are vitally necessary for both the anesthesiology and surgical teams. According to the American Society of Anesthesiologists, the interview should include, at a minimum, assessment for predisposing risk factors that contribute to increased risk of volume regurgitation, including[16] the following:

- Gastroesophageal reflux disease
- Esophageal dysmotility
- Difficulty swallowing
- Diabetes
- Gas bloat or other signs of delayed gastric emptying
- Obstructing cancer causing stasis within the esophagus

Preoperative Fasting

Preoperative fasting also is critical. Current recommendations from the American Society of Anesthesiologists Committee on Standards and Practice Parameters[16] allow the following:

- Consumption of a light meal or nonhuman milk up to 6 hours before elective procedures
- Clear liquids up to 2 hours before elective procedures (eg, water, clear tea, carbonated beverages, pulpless fruit juice, and black coffee)

These recommendations are based on studies that show that clear liquid intake in the 2 to 4 hours before induction of anesthesia was associated with a lower gastric residual volume than fasting more than 4 hours, although the differences in volume were clinically insignificant.[17] Summarized in a Cochrane review in 2003, the investigators concluded that there was no evidence supporting the standard "nil by mouth from midnight" fasting compared with a shortened fluid fast (2–4 hours) and encouraged providers to consider shorter periods of clear liquid fasting. For the thoracic surgeon, however, it is critical to note that these recommendations were accompanied by a very important caveat: there are few to no data available regarding the appropriate preoperative fasting times in populations that are considered to be at increased risk of anesthesia-related regurgitation and aspiration. Conditions such as large paraesophageal hernia, achalasia, and obstructing esophageal cancers warrant consideration of several days of clear or full liquid diet, given the poor emptying and likelihood of retained solid food matter that accompany these conditions.

Preemptive Nasogastric Tube Placement

Preemptive nasogastric tube placement has been proposed as an option for reducing aspiration risk at the time of induction. However, evidence to support this practice is lacking. There are no prospective and/or randomized data evaluating the efficacy of preemptive nasogastric tube placement and limited retrospective data. Mellin-Olsen and colleagues[18] retrospectively reviewed more than 85,000 anesthetics over a 5-year time frame and identified 25 cases of pulmonary aspiration. Aspiration events were 4 times more likely in emergency procedures and all occurred in patients receiving general anesthesia. They found no evidence to support routine preoperative gastric emptying, even in emergency cases, except for patients with suspected ileus/obstruction.[18] As such, use of a nasogastric tube should be determined by the operating surgeon and the anesthesiologist based on the patient's condition and the factors necessitating operation. Careful consideration of the risks and benefits should be undertaken, as placement of the nasogastric tube may actually contribute to vomiting and subsequent aspiration in some patients. In addition, nasogastric tube insertion in patients undergoing esophageal surgery carries high risk for injury, particularly in patients with incarcerated, obstructed paraesophageal hernia or obstructing esophageal cancer. In these cases, the surgeon should be consulted or, optimally, be present in the room during the induction of anesthesia to provide immediate guidance to the anesthesia team. Obviously, if a nasogastric tube is already in place, suctioning of the stomach should be performed.[9]

Histamine Blockers, Proton Pump Inhibitors, and Prokinetics

Histamine (H_2) antagonists, such as cimetidine, famotidine, nizatidine, and ranitidine, and proton pump inhibitors (PPIs), such as dexlansoprazole, esomeprazole, lansoprazole, omeprazole, pantoprazole, and rabeprazole, have been shown to be effective in increasing the pH and reducing the volume of gastric contents. Prokinetics, such as domperidone, metoclopramide, erythromycin, and renzapride, promote gastric emptying and in turn should reduce the risk of aspiration.[19] This theory, however, is not supported by a large amount of quality evidence. Puig and colleagues[20] evaluated the efficacy of H_2-receptor antagonists and PPIs for reducing aspiration risk in a meta-analysis of the literature in 2012. Eighteen studies were identified. Aspiration risk was defined in all but one study as a gastric pH below 2.5 and gastric volume above 25 mL. The data revealed a nonsignificant trend toward H_2-receptor antagonists being more effective than PPIs. When given as a single, oral dose immediately before operation, the H_2-receptor antagonist was significantly more effective, whereas 2 doses or intravenous dosing was similarly effective between the 2 drugs. It should be noted that the endpoint for these studies (gastric pH and gastric volume) are surrogates for the clinically important endpoint of pulmonary aspiration and that the efficacy of premedication for reduction in actual aspiration events is unproven. In addition, it is important to remember that increasing the pH of gastric contents does not completely eradicate aspiration pneumonitis. Milk and bile have been shown to do as much damage to the respiratory track as gastric contents.[9] In the current guidelines from the American Society of Anesthesiologists, routine use of gastrointestinal stimulants (eg, metoclopramide), gastric acid secretion blockers (eg, famotidine, ranitidine, omeprazole), antacids, antiemetics, and anticholinergic agents to reduce the risk of pulmonary aspiration are not recommended.[16]

Rapid-Sequence Induction

Kluger and Short[13] evaluated the timing of regurgitation and aspiration during anesthesia and found that the vast majority of events occurred during induction of anesthesia; a smaller proportion occurred during the maintenance phase of anesthesia and during emergence from anesthesia. As such, it is critically important for surgeons and anesthesiologists to have an algorithm for minimizing aspiration events in patients who are deemed high risk. One approach is to use RSI, a method of anesthesia induction that was developed to quickly achieve a protected airway in emergency or high-risk cases while minimizing risk of aspiration of regurgitated gastric contents.

The technique for RSI includes the following:

- Preoxygenation
- Rapid administration of induction and paralytic agents that are not titrated to effect
- Cricoid pressure (originally described but not currently recommended for all patients)
- Avoidance of bag and mask ventilation
- Transoral insertion of an endotracheal tube using direct or video laryngoscopy

Although theoretically appealing, the impact of RSI on prevention of aspiration, which is the reason that RSI is performed, is unclear. This is, in part, because aspiration is a rare event and would require very large numbers of patients to determine whether there was a difference in aspiration rates with and without RSI. In addition, the definition of RSI varies widely and there is not a single, universally applied, technique, which makes comparisons between studies challenging.[21] This question was examined by systematic literature review in 2007.[3] Despite reviewing 184 eligible studies, including 163 randomized controlled trials, the article concluded that the literature was insufficient to determine whether RSI reduces aspiration during induction of anesthesia. The investigators also examined the evidence for use of cricoid pressure; there were no data to support the routine use of cricoid pressure and many studies showed that the esophagus is displaced relative to the cricoid in 50% or more of patients while deforming the cricoid and obstructing the airway in 90% and 50% of patients, respectively.[22] Based on the available literature, the systematic review concluded that cricoid pressure is a benign practice and should be used in RSI, but lowered or released if the pressure is creating difficulties securing the airway.[3,23]

Patient Positioning During Induction

The optimal patient position to minimize aspiration continues to be refined. Takenaka and colleagues[24] hypothesized that airway contamination by regurgitated gastric contents could be minimized by combining use of a head-down tilt and optimizing the relationship between the head and neck. They performed a prospective study, initially in manikins with colored fluid in the esophagus and then in 30 adult volunteers. They examined aspiration events associated with combinations of a head-down tilt between 0°and 50° in 5° increments and 4 head-neck positions (neutral, simple extension, sniffing, and the Sellick position). They found that a head-down tilt that leveled the mouth with the larynx was necessary to completely prevent aspiration. More than 45° of head-down tilt was required for complete prevention of aspiration with the head-neck in the neutral position and more than 35° was needed when simple extension was used. When examined in the healthy volunteers with normal cervical spine, leveling of the mouth with the larynx was achieved with a head-down tilt of less than 15° in 87% of patients. From these findings, they concluded that a head-down tilt of 15° to 20°, combined with the Sellick position for the head to neck orientation, was optimal for minimizing tracheal and bronchial aspiration. They cautioned that intubation using the Sellick position can be challenging, and is contraindicated in patients with cervical spine instability. Their findings, however, provide support for optimizing patient positioning such that regurgitated contents are directed away from the larynx.

Others have examined lateral positioning for patients at risk for aspiration. This position is commonly used for esophageal procedures performed under monitored anesthesia and facilitates movement of regurgitated contents away from the airway. Unfortunately, most anesthesiologists have limited experience with intubating patients in this position, rendering it less useful for procedures requiring general anesthesia. Indeed, McCaul and colleagues[25] examined airway management with lateral positioning in a randomized controlled trial and found that the laryngoscopic airway examination deteriorated in 35% of patients. Lateral positioning failed to improve the laryngoscopic examination for any patient. This was most pronounced in patients undergoing endotracheal intubation when compared with laryngeal mask anesthesia. As such, although lateral positioning may optimize the orientation between the airway and the mouth and, thus, minimize aspiration, it is probably not a useful position for induction of anesthesia in most thoracic surgery patients.

MANAGEMENT OF ACUTE INTRAOPERATIVE ASPIRATION

Successful intraoperative management of pulmonary aspiration requires a high index of suspicion and immediate response. The first step in successful management of an intraoperative aspiration is the immediate recognition of gastric content in the oropharynx or the airways. Additional signs of potential aspiration include persistent hypoxia, high airway pressures, bronchospasm, and abnormal breath sounds after intubation. It is optimal if the gastric contents are visualized in the oropharynx or passing into the airway during intubation, as this allows for immediate suctioning before application of positive-pressure ventilation. In one study, 70% of the intraoperative aspiration events were confirmed by clinical visualization of regurgitation and airway penetration of the regurgitated material.[2] In this setting, the patient should be positioned with the head down and rotated laterally if possible. Orotracheal and endotracheal suctioning is indicated, either before or after orotracheal intubation, depending on whether regurgitation continues and if the airway is visible. It is recommended that the airway be secured as rapidly as possible to prevent further soilage and to facilitate airway clearance.[2] Flexible bronchoscopy is an important adjunct to orotracheal and endotracheal suctioning; indeed, having a flexible bronchoscope ready for use in patients who are known to be high risk preoperatively is warranted for airway clearance should gastric regurgitation occur. If particulate matter is present in the airway, rigid bronchoscopy may be required. There are also advocates for use of steep Trendelenburg positioning after administration of paralytics and before insertion of the laryngoscope, with Yankauer suction immediately available. In theory, regurgitated gastric contents would flow away from the airway and, given that the patient is paralyzed and cannot inhale, minimize spillage into the trachea.

The decision to proceed with the operation is at the surgeon's and anesthesiologist's discretion. Factors influencing the decision include the urgency of the operation, the patient's oxygen saturation and pulmonary compliance, and response to interventions such as bronchodilators and positive end-expiratory pressure. Antibiotics and steroid use should be individualized to the patient and are not recommended for routine use. Maintenance of mechanical ventilation also should be dictated by the usual parameters and the concern for development of ARDS based on the volume of the aspirated contents, which is associated with the likelihood of postoperative pulmonary complications.[5]

In cases of severe aspiration, cardiopulmonary arrest can occur. In these situations, cardiopulmonary resuscitation should be immediately instituted, an orotracheal airway placed, and airway clearance maneuvers performed. Early institution of extracorporeal membrane oxygenation (ECMO), if available, may provide a necessary bridge to stabilize the patient and assess potential for lung recovery. There are no published studies to date regarding the success of this strategy in adults who suffer immediate cardiac arrest subsequent to massive aspiration, and recovery in this setting is highly unlikely. Based on studies of ECMO for ARDS in adults,[26–28] a theoretic benefit for patients who subsequently develop ARDS secondary to intraoperative aspiration may exist. The decision to implement ECMO in this situation depends on the availability of ECMO, the reversibility of the underlying disease process, and the severity of associated comorbid conditions.[28]

SUMMARY

Acute intraoperative aspiration is a potentially fatal complication with significant associated morbidity. Patients undergoing thoracic surgery are at increased risk for anesthesia-related aspiration, largely due to the predisposing conditions associated with this complication. Awareness of the risk factors, predisposing conditions, maneuvers to decrease risk, and immediate management options by both the thoracic surgeon and the anesthesia team is imperative to reducing risk and optimizing patient outcomes associated with acute intraoperative pulmonary aspiration. Based on the root-cause analyses (presented previously in this article) that many of the aspiration events can be traced back to provider factors, having an experienced anesthesiologist present for high-risk cases is also critical.

ACKNOWLEDGMENTS

Imani Herring, an undergraduate at Brown University, made substantial contributions to this article.

REFERENCES

1. Jenkins K, Baker AB. Consent and anaesthetic risk. Anaesthesia 2003;58(10):962–84.
2. Kluger MT, Visvanathan T, Myburgh JA, et al. Crisis management during anaesthesia: regurgitation, vomiting, and aspiration. Qual Saf Health Care 2005;14(3):e4.
3. Neilipovitz DT, Crosby ET. No evidence for decreased incidence of aspiration after rapid sequence induction. Can J Anaesth 2007;54(9):748–64.
4. Olsson GL, Hallen B, Hambraeus-Jonzon K. Aspiration during anaesthesia: a computer-aided study of 185 358 anaesthetics. Acta Anaesthesiol Scand 1986;30(1):84–92.
5. Sakai T, Planinsic RM, Quinlan JJ, et al. The incidence and outcome of perioperative pulmonary aspiration in a university hospital: a 4-year retrospective analysis. Anesth Analg 2006;103(4):941–7.
6. Marik PE. Aspiration pneumonitis and aspiration pneumonia. N Engl J Med 2001;344(9):665–71.
7. Engelhardt T, Webster NR. Pulmonary aspiration of gastric contents in anaesthesia. Br J Anaesth 1999;83(3):453–60.
8. Janda M, Scheeren TW, Noldge-Schomburg GF. Management of pulmonary aspiration. Best Pract Res Clin Anaesthesiol 2006;20(3):409–27.
9. Benington S, Severn A. Preventing aspiration and regurgitation. Anaesth Intensive Care Med 2007;8(9):368–72.
10. Adnet F, Baud F. Relation between Glasgow coma scale and aspiration pneumonia. Lancet 1996;348(9020):123–4.
11. Irwin RS, Rippe JM. Irwin and Rippe's intensive care medicine. 7th edition. Philadelphia: Wolters Kluwer/Lippincott Williams & Wilkins Health; 2011.
12. Warner MA, Warner ME, Weber JG. Clinical significance of pulmonary aspiration during the perioperative period. Anesthesiology 1993;78(1):56–62.
13. Kluger MT, Short TG. Aspiration during anaesthesia: a review of 133 cases from the Australian Anaesthetic Incident Monitoring Study (AIMS). Anaesthesia 1999;54(1):19–26.
14. Klanarong S, Suksompong S, Hintong T, et al. Perioperative pulmonary aspiration: an analysis of 28 reports from the Thai Anesthesia Incident Monitoring Study (Thai AIMS). J Med Assoc Thai 2011;94(4):457–64.
15. Nafiu OO, Bradin S, Tremper KK. Knowledge, attitude, and practice regarding cricoid pressure of ED personnel at a large US teaching hospital. J Emerg Nurs 2009;35(1):11–5.
16. American Society of Anesthesiologists Committee. Practice guidelines for preoperative fasting and the use of pharmacologic agents to reduce the risk of pulmonary aspiration: application to healthy patients undergoing elective procedures: an updated report by the American Society of Anesthesiologists Committee on Standards and Practice Parameters. Anesthesiology 2011;114(3):495–511.
17. Brady M, Kinn S, Stuart P. Preoperative fasting for adults to prevent perioperative complications. Cochrane Database Syst Rev 2003;(4):CD004423.
18. Mellin-Olsen J, Fasting S, Gisvold SE. Routine preoperative gastric emptying is seldom indicated. A study of 85,594 anaesthetics with special focus on aspiration pneumonia. Acta Anaesthesiol Scand 1996;40(10):1184–8.
19. Clark K, Lam LT, Gibson S, et al. The effect of ranitidine versus proton pump inhibitors on gastric secretions: a meta-analysis of randomised control trials. Anaesthesia 2009;64(6):652–7.
20. Puig I, Calzado S, Suarez D, et al. Meta-analysis: comparative efficacy of H2-receptor antagonists and proton pump inhibitors for reducing aspiration risk during anaesthesia depending on the administration route and schedule. Pharm Res 2012;65(4):480–90.

21. Ehrenfeld JM, Cassedy EA, Forbes VE, et al. Modified rapid sequence induction and intubation: a survey of United States current practice. Anesth Analg 2012;115(1):95–101.
22. Boet S, Duttchen K, Chan J, et al. Cricoid pressure provides incomplete esophageal occlusion associated with lateral deviation: a magnetic resonance imaging study. J Emerg Med 2012;42(5):606–11.
23. Butler J, Sen A. Towards evidence-based emergency medicine: best BETs from the Manchester Royal Infirmary. BET 1: cricoid pressure in emergency rapid sequence induction. Emerg Med J 2013;30(2):163–5.
24. Takenaka I, Aoyama K, Iwagaki T. Combining head-neck position and head-down tilt to prevent pulmonary aspiration of gastric contents during induction of anaesthesia: a volunteer and manikin study. Eur J Anaesthesiol 2012;29(8):380–5.
25. McCaul CL, Harney D, Ryan M, et al. Airway management in the lateral position: a randomized controlled trial. Anesth Analg 2005;101(4):1221–5 [table of contents].
26. Peek GJ, Mugford M, Tiruvoipati R, et al. Efficacy and economic assessment of conventional ventilatory support versus extracorporeal membrane oxygenation for severe adult respiratory failure (CESAR): a multicentre randomised controlled trial. Lancet 2009;374(9698):1351–63.
27. Chang WW, Tsai FC, Tsai TY, et al. Predictors of mortality in patients successfully weaned from extracorporeal membrane oxygenation. PLoS One 2012; 7(8):e42687.
28. Turner DA, Cheifetz IM. Extracorporeal membrane oxygenation for adult respiratory failure. Respir Care 2013;58(6):1038–52.

Coagulopathy and Anticoagulation During Thoracic Surgery

Mathew Thomas, MD[a,*], K. Robert Shen, MD[b]

KEYWORDS

- Perioperative anticoagulation • Perioperative antithrombotics • Perioperative antiplatelets
- Bleeding • Thromboembolism

KEY POINTS

- Anticoagulation and antiplatelet medications can cause severe bleeding during any major surgery.
- Little evidence exists to guide the optimal perioperative management of antithrombotic medications in thoracic surgery.
- Assessment of the risks of bleeding and thromboembolism in individual patients is the most important determinant of whether to continue or stop antithrombotic medications perioperatively.
- Multidisciplinary decision making and patient communication are essential to ensure best outcomes.

INTRODUCTION

Most noncardiac thoracic procedures have the potential to cause major bleeding as a result of vascular injury or diffuse bleeding from the chest wall, mediastinum, or lung. Procedures involving extensive dissection, such as pleural adhesiolysis, pleurectomy, lung decortication, or mechanical pleurodesis, can be associated with significant loss of blood. The risk of surgical bleeding may be compounded by the presence of drugs that affect hemostasis, such as anticoagulation or antiplatelet agents. As a precaution against excessive bleeding, these antithrombotic medications are often temporarily interrupted during the perioperative period, which in turn increases the risk of thromboembolic events.[1] Surgery alone promotes coagulation with the release of multiple procoagulant factors[2] and is recognized as a major risk factor for recurrent venous thromboembolism (VTE).[3,4] The significant complications that can occur from either cessation or continuation of these medications during the perioperative period makes it imperative for every surgeon to be well aware of their pharmacologic properties and to have a well-formulated plan for their perioperative management.

Anticoagulation therapy is used in the setting of either arterial thromboembolism (ATE) or VTE, with more fatalities and disabilities associated with the former condition.[5] The most common indications for chronic anticoagulation include mechanical heart valves, chronic atrial fibrillation, and a history of VTE.[6] Antiplatetets are used primarily in patients with coronary stents, peripheral arterial stents, or peripheral vascular disease. The number of patients in North America who are on an antithrombotic drug and require an intervention that can cause major bleeding is estimated to be approximately 250,000 annually.[6] Although guidelines for the perioperative management of antithrombotic medications have been established by many

The authors have nothing to disclose.
[a] Division of Cardiothoracic Surgery, Mayo Clinic, 4500 San Pablo Road, Jacksonville, FL 32082, USA; [b] Division of General Thoracic Surgery, Mayo Clinic, 200 First Street Southwest, Rochester, MN 55205, USA
* Corresponding author.
E-mail address: thomas.mathew@mayo.edu

Thorac Surg Clin 25 (2015) 309–323
http://dx.doi.org/10.1016/j.thorsurg.2015.04.005
1547-4127/15/$ – see front matter

medical societies, these recommendations are followed in only 16% to 31% of patients, with a large percentage of patients either under- or overtreated with bridging therapy.[7,8]

The optimal perioperative management of antithrombotics has always been controversial and is now even more challenging with the recent introduction of newer antithrombotic agents. Unfortunately, in the absence of any level A evidence (multiple randomized controlled studies) that evaluates the effect of antithrombotic drugs in the perioperative setting, most current society guidelines are expert opinions based largely on observational studies, with recommendation grades ranging from 1C to 2C.[6,9–11] The most recent antithrombotic guidelines, 9th edition (AT9) by the American College of Chest Physicians (ACCP) have fewer recommendations than the previous editions due to the elimination of those not backed by strong evidence.[6] Given the paucity of robust evidence to direct the perioperative management of antithrombotic therapy, creation of institution-specific standardized protocols may be the most appropriate way to ensure the best outcomes.[6,12–14]

CLASSIFICATION OF ANTICOAGULATION AGENTS

Major Classification

Until recently, the 3 major classes of anticoagulants were the oral vitamin K antagonists (VKAs), parenteral heparin, and parenteral direct thrombin inhibitors. Over the past decade, several oral anticoagulants were introduced into the market, leading to the creation of a fourth class, novel oral anticoagulants (NOACs).

1. Oral VKAs

   Oral VKAs include warfarin and other coumarol derivatives, such as acenocoumarol and phenprocoumon. Warfarin is perhaps the most common long-term oral anticoagulation agent used, although it is being gradually replaced by NOACs. Warfarin activity is measured by the international normalized ratio (INR), which usually returns to normal (<1.5) after 5 days of drug cessation. There is insufficient evidence to determine the safe level of INR required for major surgery, although an INR greater than or equal to 2.0 has been generally assumed to increase bleeding risk.[6]

2. Parenteral heparin

   The 2 common forms of parenteral heparin are unfractionated heparin (UFH) and the low-molecular-weight heparins (LMWHs). LMWH can be administered subcutaneously (SC) once or twice daily in the outpatient setting, whereas intravenous (IV) UFH requires admission to the hospital.[1] Although commonly used for bridging, the Food and Drug Administration (FDA) does not currently approve LMWH for this purpose. Both LMWH and UFH have approximately equal times of onset of anticoagulation (1 hour), with peak activity seen at approximately 3 to 6 hours. UFH has a dose-dependent half-life of 30 to 120 minutes and can be rapidly reversed. It is suitable for use in patients with renal insufficiency because the dosing is not affected by renal clearance.

3. Parenteral direct thrombin inhibitors

   Argatroban and bilvalirudin are 2 IV drugs in this class that are reserved for use when heparin is contraindicated, such as in heparin-induced thrombocytopenia.

4. NOACs

   Disadvantages of VKA therapy led to the development of alternative oral anticoagulation agents, which continue to be introduced to the market. These drugs are commonly referred to as NOACs or direct oral anticoagulants (DOACs) but have varying sites of action in the coagulation cascade. Compared with VKAs, NOACs do not require frequent monitoring or interact with food and most medications, have shorter half-lives, and have demonstrated equivalent benefit for specific conditions. They have a rapid onset of action with the maximum effect seen in approximately 3 hours after intake.

   Although NOACs have made chronic anticoagulation therapy more patient friendly, they have also introduced fresh challenges with regard to their perioperative management; these include the lack of standard monitoring methods or specific antidotes to rapidly reverse their effects for emergent surgery or major bleeding. Without standard guidelines or long-term data to guide the perioperative management of NOACs, the operating surgeon and the prescribing physician may make conflicting recommendations favoring what each considers is the greater risk (ie, bleeding or thromboembolism).

Classification of Novel Oral Anticoagulants

1. Direct thrombin inhibitors (**Table 1**)

   Dabigatran is an FDA-approved NOAC that directly inhibits both free and fibrin-bound thrombin without using antithrombin.

Table 1
Properties of novel oral anticoagulants

Classification Based on Mechanism of Action	Drug	Peak Onset of Action	Half-Life	Plasma Protein Binding (%)	Renal Excretion (%)	Antidote	Laboratory Tests to Monitor Activity[a]	Suggested Strategies for Emergent Reversal
Direct thrombin inhibitor	Dabigatran	1.25–3 h	12–17 h	35	80	None	dTT—Hemoclot assay dTT >65 may be associated with an increased risk of bleeding; aPTT	Dialysis, fab, activated charcoal (within 2 h of intake), PCC
Factor Xa inhibitor	Rivaroxaban	2–4 h	5–9 h	92–95	66	None	Factor Xa activity assays; PT	PCC, activated charcoal (within 2 h of intake)
	Apixaban	3–4 h	8–15 h	87	25	None	Factor Xa activity assays; PT	PCC, activated charcoal (within 2–6 h of intake)

Abbreviations: aPT, activated prothrombin time; dTT, diluted thrombin time; fab, fully humanized antibody fragment; PCC, prothrombin complex concentrates; PT, prothrombin time.

[a] There are no standard monitoring tests for NOACs.

2. Factor Xa inhibitors (see **Table 1**)
   Factor Xa is a rate-limiting factor in the coagulation pathway; drugs that inhibit it directly without the need for antithrombin are used in the treatment of VTE. Rivaroxaban and apixaban are 2 such drugs approved for use in the United States, Europe, and Canada, whereas a third drug, edoxaban is awaiting FDA approval as of this writing. Prothrombin complex concentrates (PCCs) have been shown to neutralize rivaroxaban in patients with major bleeding.[15] Bebulin (factors II, IX, and X) and Kcentra (II, VII, IX, X, and proteins C and S) are 2 PCCs that are now commercially available for use.[16]

CLASSIFICATION OF ANTIPLATELET AGENTS

Drugs that primarily affect hemostasis by interfering with platelet functions are commonly classified based on their mechanism of action (**Table 2**).

1. Cyclooxygenase (COX) inhibitors
   COX inhibitors may be reversible or nonreversible inhibitors. Aspirin (acetylsalicylic acid [ASA]) is the only nonreversible drug in this class used specifically for its antiplatelet properties. Nonsteroidal anti-inflammatory drugs reversibly inhibit COX pathways and may affect bleeding during surgery but are not used for antiplatelet therapy.
2. ADP receptor/P_2Y_{12} receptor blockers
   Clopidogrel, the most commonly used drug in this class has irreversible antiplatelet activity. Ticagrelor is a reversible P_2Y_{12} receptor blocker.
3. GP IIb/IIIa antagonists
   Abciximab, tirofiban, and eptifibatide are IV administered, reversible competitors of the GP IIb/IIIa receptors used for short-term antiplatelet therapy.
4. Phosphodiesterase inhibitors
   Phosphodiesterase inhibitors (eg, dipyridamole and cilostazol) have both vasodilator and reversible antiplatelet activities.

ASSESSMENT OF RISK

The most important determinant in perioperatively managing antithrombotic drugs is the balance between the risk of major surgical bleeding with continued antithrombotic therapy and the risk of thromboembolic events when antithrombotic therapy is held.[6] This is best assessed jointly by the operating surgeon (bleeding risk) and the practitioner responsible for prescribing the antithrombotic therapy (thromboembolic risk), such as the cardiologist, vascular medicine specialist or vascular surgeon, neurosurgeon, neurointerventionalist, and so forth. Communication between the vested parties, including the patient, is critical in ensuring that the best practices are followed.[11]

Multiple scoring methods have been proposed to determine the risks of thromboembolic events or bleeding with chronic anticoagulation. There are currently no validated scoring methods, however, to directly compare the bleeding risks during major surgery while on antithrombotic agents and predict the risks of thromboembolic events when these drugs are temporarily discontinued.

Risk of Thromboembolism

It is important to distinguish the risk of recurrent VTE due to cessation of chronic anticoagulation from the general risk of postoperative VTE. The risk of systemic (arterial) thromboembolism versus the risk of VTE should also be distinguished, because there are considerable differences in complications and effectiveness of anticoagulation in these conditions.

Risk Stratification

Based on the general estimated annual risk (AR) for thromboembolism, patients may be classified as high risk (>10% AR), moderate risk (5%–10% AR), or low risk (<5% AR) for thromboembolic events (**Box 1**).

A prior history of thromboembolism, chronic atrial fibrillation, mechanical mitral valve, older-generation aortic valves, greater than 1 mechanical valve, hypercoagulable conditions, or left ventricular ejection fraction (LVEF) less than 30% confers the highest risk for thromboembolic events.[17,18] These classifications, however, are by no means absolute and individual patients may fall into one risk category or another depending on the assessment method used.

Risk Scores

Perhaps the most well-known scoring method for the risk of ATE is the CHADS score and its subsequent modifications, including $CHADS_2$ and CHA_2DS_2-VASc (congestive heart failure, hypertension, age $\geq$75 years [2 points], diabetes mellitus, stroke or TIA [2 points], vascular disease, age 65 to 74, and sex category [female gender]) for patients with atrial fibrillation.[19,20] Although an average risk of systemic embolization of 4.5% per year in all patients with nonvalvular atrial fibrillation has been reported, risk scores give a better estimate of the individual risk, which may vary from 1% to 20%.[21–25]

Table 2
Classification of antiplatelet drugs

Classification Based on Mechanism of Action	Reversibility	Commonly Prescribed Drugs	Time to Onset of Action After Intake	Time to Restoration of Normal Platelet Function After Last Dose	Antidotes	Suggested Strategies for Emergent Reversal
COX inhibitors	Nonreversible	ASA	Minutes	7–10 d	None	Desmopressin, platelet transfusion
ADP receptor/P_2Y_{12} receptor blockers	Nonreversible	Clopidogrel Ticlopidine Prasugrel	1–2 h[a]	5–7 d 10–14 d 5–9 d	None	Desmopressin, platelet transfusion
	Reversible	Ticagrelor	1–4 h	5–7 d	None	Desmopressin, platelet transfusion
GP IIb/IIIa antagonists	Reversible	Abciximab Tirofiban Eptifibatide	10–30 min	12–48 h 4–8 h	None	Stop medication; Desmopressin, platelet ± cryoprecipitate transfusion; hemodialysis (tirofiban, eptifibatide)
Phosphodiesterase inhibitors	Reversible	Dipyridamole Cilostazol	75 min 2–12 wk	48–96 h	None	Desmopressin, platelet transfusion

[a] Dose dependent.

Box 1
Risk stratification

Venous thromboembolism

- High risk: VTE less than 3 months, severe thrombophilia
- Moderate risk: VTE 3–12 months, nonsevere thrombophilia, recurrent VTE, active cancer
- Low risk: VTE greater than 12 months

Arterial thromboembolism

- High risk: MV prosthesis, older-generation AV prosthesis, recent stroke/TIA (3–6 months), $CHADS_2$ 5–6, CHA_2DS_2-VASc score $\geq$2; valvular afibrillation, left ventricular dysfunction [LVEF <30%])
- Moderate risk: BLAVP + $\geq$1 risk factors (afibrillation, prior stroke/TIA, hypertension, diabetes, CHF, age >75 y); $CHADS_2$ 3–4, CHA_2DS_2-VASc 1
- Low risk: BLAVP without risk factors; $CHADS_2$ 0–2, CHA_2DS_2-VASc 0

Abbreviations: AV, aortic valve; BLAVP, bileaflet aortic valve prosthesis; CHF, congestive heart failure; MV, mitral valve replacement; TIA, transient ischemic attack.

Data from Douketis JD, Spyropoulos AC, Spencer FA, et al. Perioperative management of antithrombotic therapy: antithrombotic therapy and prevention of thrombosis, 9th ed: American College of Chest Physicians evidence-based clinical practice guidelines. Chest 2012;141(2 Suppl):e326S–50S; and Fleisher LA, Fleischmann KE, Auerbach AD, et al. 2014 ACC/AHA guideline on perioperative cardiovascular evaluation and management of patients undergoing noncardiac surgery: a report of the American College of Cardiology/American Heart Association Task Force on Practice Guidelines. J Am Coll Cardiol 2014;64(22):e77–137.

Scoring systems for VTE (eg, D-dimer, age, sex, and hormone therapy [DASH])[26] have also been described but have not been as popular as ATE scores. Clinical history is critical in determining the risk of recurrent VTE; a history of unprovoked VTE significantly increases the risk of recurrence when anticoagulation is discontinued, regardless of the duration of treatment prior to discontinuation.[27] Active malignancy is well known to increase the risks for both VTE and periprocedural bleeding in anticoagulated patients.[28] The rate of major bleeding is also higher in chronically anticoagulated patients with active cancer who have periprocedural bridging with heparin.[28] These important points should be kept in mind because the majority of noncardiac thoracic surgery is performed in patients with active malignancies.

Timing

The risk of recurrent VTE does not remain constant with time after the initial event. The first 3 months (50% risk), especially within the first 30 days (40% risk) after a VTE has occurred, is the period with the greatest risk of recurrence.[5,29] Discontinuation of anticoagulation during the first 3 months increases the risk of recurrent VTE significantly by approximately 100-fold,[5] and elective procedures should be avoided during this time period. An exception to this observation is seen in patients with active malignancies who have had a VTE, because they remain at an increased risk of a recurrence regardless of the time from the initial event.

Timing is also an important factor to be considered in patients with coronary and peripheral arterial stents who require surgery. Repair of arterial endothelial damage caused by placement of the stent is a prothrombotic process and is most active during the first 6 weeks but does not completely stop after that. Stent thrombosis is most likely to occur if antiplatelet therapy is held less than 6 weeks after stents have been placed. The kind of stent placed also determines the safe time period to hold antiplatelet therapy because drug-eluting stents (DESs) require longer times to heal than bare metal stents (BMSs). Perioperative management of stents is described in greater detail later.

Risk of Bleeding

Classification of bleeding

Although it is difficult to preoperatively quantify the risk of bleeding, an experienced operating surgeon can estimate the risk of major bleeding (commonly defined as $\geq$2 L)[9,22] for an intended procedure. Most major thoracic surgical operations are considered high risk for major bleeding whereas percutaneous procedures, such as needle biopsies, are generally considered minimal risk in various society guidelines. Such categorizations are too generalized, however, and based on heterogenous groups of patients to be of any real value in understanding the effects of antithrombotic medications or the proper timing for stopping and resuming them perioperatively.[30] The hypervascular nature of the lung and the potential for severe bleeding even with a simple needle biopsy should never be disregarded. The presence of antithrombotic therapy may lead to severe bleeding in procedures that normally cause minimal bleeding.

Risk scores

Similar to risk scores for thromboembolism, bleeding scores for patients on anticoagulation have been devised but are not commonly used, probably due to their unreliability.[31,32] One such scoring method is HAS-BLED (hypertension, abnormal renal or liver function, stroke, bleeding history or predisposition, labile INR, elderly [>65 years], and concomitant usage of drugs/alcohol) score, which estimates the risk of bleeding during intervention in patients on chronic anticoagulation and also during bridging in atrial fibrillation patients.[8,33] The value of such scores in determining perioperative antithrombotic management for major surgery is unclear.

In patients with a prior history of excessive bleeding during procedures or a family history of bleeding, a complete work-up for hematologic disorders should be performed.[34] To the best of the authors' knowledge, no data are currently available to determine if patients with a personal or family history of abnormal bleeding require a longer period of preoperative cessation of chronic antithrombotic medication.

Risk of Bleeding Versus Venous Thromboembolism

In a study of 775 chronically anticoagulated patients with VTE referred to the Mayo Clinic Thrombophilia Center over a 10-year period for periprocedural anticoagulation management,[35] patients were classified based on their risk for recurrent VTE, depending on which pre- and postoperative bridging with TD LMWH was performed. They were then followed for 3 months afterward, during which the cumulative major bleeding ($\geq$2 units packed red blood cell transfusion or $\geq$2 g drop in hemoglobin; or intracranial, intraspinal, intraocular, retroperitoneal, pericardial, or fatal bleeding) and thromboembolism rates were reported to be 1.8% each. Active cancer was the only independent predictor of major hemorrhage, recurrent thrombosis, and death in that study. The investigators of the study concluded that the incidence of recurrent thromboembolism, major bleeding, and death after periprocedural discontinuation of anticoagulation therapy for VTE is low.

In another larger multicenter prospective study that included 1262 patients on chronic anticoagulation for all causes who were bridged with LMWH and followed for 30 days after their procedures, thromboembolism and major hemorrhage rates were 0.4% and 1.2%, respectively.[36] This study included a heterogenous population of patients and a wide spectrum of procedures, hence cannot be used to deduct specifically the effect on major surgical procedures.

GENERAL PRINCIPLES OF PERIOPERATIVE ANTITHROMBOTIC MANAGEMENT

Multisociety guidelines for perioperative management of antithrombotic medication[6,11] are based on the following broad principles:

- Elective procedures that have a major risk of bleeding with antithrombotic medication should be scheduled at a time that allows complete metabolism of the drug from the system prior to the operation.
- When risk of VTE from stopping chronic anticoagulation is considered significant enough, bridging therapy should be instituted and the short-acting anticoagulation drug discontinued at the shortest possible interval that keeps bleeding risk at a minimum.
- Antithrombotic therapy should be reinstituted at the earliest possible time postoperatively, when considered safe.
- It is important to discuss the risks of perioperative bleeding and thromboembolism with the patient. The possible need for returning to the operating room to evacuate hemothorax and the potential fatal complications of VTE or thrombosis of arterial/venous stents should be clearly discussed.

A summary of the authors' review of the latest ACCP and American Heart Association (AHA)/American College of Cardiology (ACC) guidelines is in **Box 2**.

PERIOPERATIVE MANAGEMENT OF ANTICOAGULATION THERAPY

Discontinuation and Bridging of Anticoagulation Agents

Anticoagulation therapy is discontinued before surgery and for a certain duration afterward to achieve a normal coagulation profile and reduce the risk of major perioperative bleeding. Due to the increased risk of thromboembolism with this strategy, the period of subtherapeutic anticoagulation should be as short as possible.

In patients who are at high risk for developing thromboembolism, shorter-acting antithrombotics are used to decrease the at-risk time, which is known as bridging.

Box 2
Summary of AT9 & American College of Cardiology/American Heart Association antithrombotic guidelines

Perioperative anticoagulation recommendations

- Stop VKA 5 days before surgery, if indicated by risk assessment
- Bridging recommendations for anticoagulants
  - High risk—bridge
  - Low risk—no bridging
  - Intermediate risk—individualize
- Time to stop bridging before surgery
  - IV TD UFH: 4–6 h
  - SC TD LMWH: 24 h
- Resumption of anticoagulation/bridging postoperatively
  - Resume VKA 12–24 h if adequate hemostasis
  - SC LMWH for high-risk bleeding surgery: 48–72 h

Perioperative antiplatelet recommendations

- ASA therapy
  - Moderate to high risk for CVE (secondary prevention): continue perioperative ASA
  - Low risk for CVE (primary prevention): discontinue ASA 7–10 days before surgery
- Antiplatelets for coronary stents
  - Minimum time[a] to defer surgery after intervention
    - Balloon angioplasty: 2 weeks
    - BMS: AT9 6 weeks; AHA 30 days
    - DES: 6 months
  - If surgery inevitable before the recommended optimal waiting period and bleeding risk less than risk of CVE, continue DAPT.
  - If DAPT not acceptable due to high risk of bleeding, consider monotherapy with ASA; restart DAPT ASAP after surgery.

Abbreviation: CVE, cardiovascular event.

[a] The minimum time to defer surgery is the period with the highest risk of stent thrombosis when DAPT is interrupted. It is not necessarily the same as the "optimal" period to continue uninterrupted DAPT, which may be longer.

Data from Douketis JD, Spyropoulos AC, Spencer FA, et al. Perioperative management of antithrombotic therapy: antithrombotic therapy and prevention of thrombosis, 9th ed: American College of Chest Physicians evidence-based clinical practice guidelines. Chest 2012;141(2 Suppl):e326S–50S; and Fleisher LA Fleischmann KE, Auerbach AD, et al. 2014 ACC/AHA guideline on perioperative cardiovascular evaluation and management of patients undergoing noncardiac surgery: a report of the American College of Cardiology/American Heart Association Task Force on Practice Guidelines. J Am Coll Cardiol 2014;64(22):e77–137.

Definition

AT9 defines bridging anticoagulation as "the administration of a short-acting anticoagulant, consisting of subcutaneous (SC) low-molecular-weight heparin (LMWH) or IV unfractionated heparin (UFH), for an ∼ 10 to 12-day period during interruption of VKA therapy when the international normalized ratio (INR) is not within a therapeutic range."[6]

The goal of bridging is risk reduction of ATE to the cerebrovascular and systemic circulation and recurrent VTE.[6] Bridging is recommended for patients who are at high risk for thromboembolism[6,11] and not recommended for low-risk patients.[6,10,11] For moderate-risk patients, the decision whether to bridge or not should be individualized.[6,11]

LMWH or UFH dosing is commonly categorized as high-dose (therapeutic), intermediate-dose and low-dose (prophylactic).[6] Therapeutic doses (TDs) are most commonly used for the purpose of bridging (**Table 3**). In high doses, LWMH or UFH has similar thromboembolic preventive properties to VKA in patients with mechanical valves and acute VTE.[6,37] Prophylactic-dose LMWH is commonly used in the prevention of postoperative VTE but has not been shown to be efficient in preventing ATE, such as ischemic stroke in atrial fibrillation.[38,39] UFH may be more effective in this regard.[40]

The authors follow the ACCP recommendations to stop VKA 5 days before elective surgery when interruption is required,[6] aiming for an INR less than or equal to 1.5. Drugs, such as warfarin, however, may have significant interpatient variability in metabolism, and longer periods of stoppage may be necessary in certain category of patients. A prospective study of 22 patients receiving a fixed dose of warfarin and then discontinued showed wide variability of the rate of decrease of the INR over time.[41] Based on this observation, the investigators recommended at least 4 doses of warfarin to be held to achieve an INR less than 1.2, when the steady state was 2.0 to 3.0. An extremely elevated INR (>6.0), extreme age, active cancer, and decompensated heart failure are risk factors for prolonged delay in reduction of the INR.[42] In patients with these conditions, measuring the INR 24 hours prior to surgery is recommended to ensure that the expected reversal has occurred.[43] If the INR has not declined appropriately, the surgery may be delayed for a few more days; when this is not an option, oral vitamin K can be given (1 mg for an INR of 1.6 or 1.7; 2 mg for an INR >1.8) and the INR remeasured on the day of surgery.[1]

There is no consensus among different society guidelines regarding the optimal time to discontinue NOACs before major surgery, with recommendations ranging from 48 hours[11,14] to 5 days.[44] Some groups recommend discontinuation times to be based on a patient's creatinine clearance.[16] Until more evidence with regard to their perioperative management becomes available, the authors prefer to discontinue NOACs 5 days before surgery due to the absence of a specific antidote for NOAC-induced bleeding. Bridging for such patients is determined based on their risks of thromboembolism versus bleeding.[16]

The authors' preference is to start bridging when INR less than 2.0, as recommended by most guidelines, and often use SC LMWH for this purpose and IV UFH for specific patients. In the case of warfarin, the interpatient variation (discussed previously) in the normalization of the INR[41] has to be taken into account before bridging is initiated. In general, the average half-life of warfarin is approximately 22 hours and the INR usually drops to less than 2.0 approximately 60 hours after the last dose, after which bridging can be initiated.[1,41]

Discontinuation of LMWH is recommended 24 to 48 hours before surgery[1,45] due to the prolonged presence of therapeutic anti-Xa levels in greater than two-thirds of patients receiving TD LMWH. If the risk of VTE or ATE is high, the patient may have to be placed on IV TD UFH, which should then be discontinued 4 to 6 hours before surgery. The authors do not routinely measure factor Xa levels in patients bridged with LMWH prior to surgery, because there is no evidence to support such preoperative testing.

Postoperative Resumption of Anticoagulation Therapy

Postoperative risk for VTE is different from preoperative risk. A 100-fold increase in the risk of VTE after surgery is expected; hence, for patients with a less than 3-month history of prior VTE, postoperative IV UFH should be strongly considered when it is safe to start.[5] After 3 months, however, the risk drops to near normal levels and there are no data to support the use of postoperative IV UFH.

The Prospective Perioperative Enoxaparin Cohort Trial (PROSPECT) study reported an overall major perioperative bleeding rate of 3.5% with bridging therapy using TD LMWH in patients on chronic anticoagulation.[46] This study included

Table 3
Therapeutic dose heparins

Heparin Class	Therapeutic Dose	Suggested Uses
A. UFH	Dose to obtain aPTT levels 1.5–2 times normal	Atrial fibrillation; aortic mechanical valves with high risk; recent VTE (<3 mo); mechanical mitral valves
B. LMWH		
a. Enoxaparin	1 mg/kg bid or 1.5 mg/kg qd	
b. Dalteparin	100 IU/kg bid or 200 IU/kg qd	
c. Tinzaparin	175 IU/kg daily	

patients who had oral warfarin resumed the evening of postoperative day 0 and TD LMWH resumed 12 to 24 hours after surgery, provided hemostasis was achieved. Major bleeding was observed in 20% of patients who underwent major surgery of greater than 1-hour duration and in whom TD LMWH was given. None of the patients with major bleeding had undergone a thoracic operation. Based on observational studies, such as PROSPECT, most guidelines suggest resuming therapeutic anticoagulation 12 to 24 hours after surgery, if considered safe from a hemostasis perspective.[6,11,14] The authors' practice is to resume SC prophylactic heparin soon after surgery based on the assessment of bleeding risk, followed by bridging with TD LMWH 24 to 48 hours later, as outlined in the ACCP guidelines. If there is a high risk for bleeding, resumption of TD LMWH may be postponed to 48 to 72 hours after surgery.

In the absence of any evidence-backed guidelines to direct their postoperative management, the authors prefer to wait at least 72 hours before restarting NOACs. In the interval, prophylactic heparin is continued and postoperative bridging[14] instituted, as described previously.

PERIOPERATIVE MANAGEMENT OF ANTIPLATELET THERAPY

Perioperative management of antiplatelet therapy is best addressed with regard to indication for its use (ie, coronary stents, peripheral stents, cerebrovascular stents, and so forth). The most common indication, prevention of thrombosis after coronary stents, is discussed.

Discontinuation of Antiplatelet Therapy for Coronary Stents

Patients with coronary stents are not uncommonly seen for consideration of thoracic surgery. Due to the high risk of stent thrombosis, dual antiplatelet therapy (DAPT) with ASA and a second antiplatelet agent (commonly from the thienopyridine class of drugs [eg, clopidogrel and prasugrel]) is now standard of care after stent placement. These drugs significantly increase the risk of major surgical bleeding if continued perioperatively, especially when DAPT is continued.[47,48] The risk of major bleeding was found 1% higher when clopidogrel is held less than 5 days before coronary artery bypass grafting (CABG).[49] Prasugrel is associated with higher risk of major bleeding compared with clopidogrel.[50]

An estimated 4% to 11% of patients undergo noncardiac surgery in the first 2 years after stent placement.[51–53] Premature cessation of DAPT has been reported the single most important predictor of stent thrombosis, occurring in approximately 40% of patients.[54] The complications of stent thrombosis are significant, resulting in myocardial infarction in 50% to 70% and fatalities in 9% to 45% of patients.[55–57]

There are 2 main classes of coronary stents, the BMSs and the DESs. Although both are equally susceptible, DESs have a longer period of vulnerability to stent thrombosis compared with BMSs.[58,59] As a result, a longer time of up to 1 year of uninterrupted DAPT is usually recommended for DESs[11,60] but may vary between different generations. Second-generation DESs may require only 6 months of uninterrupted DAPT according to some studies.[61]

The most recent multisociety guidelines suggest waiting a minimum of 2 weeks after balloon angioplasty, 4 to 6 weeks after BMS implantation, and optimally 6 to 12 months after DES implantation before performing noncardiac surgery.[6,11,62] In patients for whom surgery cannot be delayed due to the risk of waiting longer, it may be considered 6 months after DES implantation. These guidelines also suggest that if surgery cannot be delayed until the recommended time, it should be done while continuing preferably DAPT or at least ASA monotherapy, if considered safe. It is important for patients to be made aware of the risks and benefits of performing surgery earlier than the recommended optimal waiting period.

Mortality rates are the highest when noncardiac surgery is performed within 6 weeks of coronary stent placement[63,64] and have been attributed to the increased thrombogenesis seen after surgery.[65] Major adverse cardiovascular events (MACEs) were reported in 13.3% of patients who underwent noncardiac surgery less than or equal to 1 month of BMS placement or less than 3 to 6 months after DES placement but in only 0.6% of patients who had surgery beyond those time periods.[64]

In patients who require intervention for coronary artery disease and plan to undergo noncardiac surgery within 14 to 42 days after the PCI, balloon angioplasty should be considered.[11] BMS should be considered when surgery is anticipated greater than 30 days to 1 year, and DES if surgery can be delayed for greater than 1 year. If surgery is required in less than 2 weeks, and revascularization is critical, CABG in combination with the noncardiac surgery is suggested as an option.[11]

Multisociety guidelines also recommend continuing perioperative ASA in moderate- to high-risk patients with coronary stents undergoing noncardiac surgery and in patients without stents in whom the risks of cardiac events are higher than the risk of bleeding.[6,11] Perioperative ASA monotherapy may be reasonable these patients, because it has been shown to decrease the rate of MACE[66] without necessarily increasing the rate of major bleeding.[67] In cases of low-risk patients, ASA should be stopped 7 to 10 days before surgery.

When indicated, the authors discontinue nonreversible antiplatelet agents 5 to 7 days before surgery, due to the time it takes to replenish the pool of normal platelets by the bone marrow (7–10 days).

Bridging for Antiplatelet Therapy

There are no approved bridging agents for antiplatelet therapy. Short-acting glycoprotein (GP) IIb/IIIa inhibitors, such as eptifibatide and tirofiban, have been reportedly used for bridging in some cases of extremely high-risk patients with variable results.[68,69] These medications are available as infusions and require inpatient admission. There have been no studies evaluating bridging for antiplatelet therapy; therefore, their use is not advised in the most recent guidelines.[6,11]

Resumption of Antiplatelet Therapy

There is a paucity of evidence to determine the appropriate time to resume DAPT after major surgery and, as a result, recommendations are vague even in society guidelines.[6,11] The authors usually wait 12 to 24 hours to resume antiplatelet therapy, depending on the assessment of hemostasis and the likelihood of returning to the operating room for bleeding. ASA has a rapid onset of action (within minutes) compared with clopidogrel (at a maintenance dose of 75 mg/d), which may take 5 to 10 days for maximum action to occur without a loading dose.[6]

VENA CAVAL FILTERS

Inferior or superior vena caval filters are devices used in the prevention of pulmonary embolism (PE). They are percutaneously placed and may be temporary or permanent.

Current perioperative indications for vena caval filter in patients undergoing surgery are limited to patients with less than 1-month history of VTE when anticoagulation is contraindicated.[70] Retrievable filters are recommended. Evidence to support the use of filters in other high-risk patients is sparse, and the risks and benefits in each case must be individually considered.[71,72] Caval filters in themselves are most often complicated by recurrent thrombosis,[73] which may lead to PE.[72,74]

HEREDITARY HYPERCOAGULABLE CONDITIONS

Patients with genetically acquired hypercoagulability disorders, such as factor V Leiden mutation or antiphospholipid antibody (aPL), have an increased risk of thrombosis during surgery, even in the presence of anticoagulation.[75–77] Deep venous thrombosis and cerebrovascular embolization are the 2 most common manifestations of thromboembolic disease in the aPL population, whereas VTE without systemic embolization seems to be the hallmark for factor V Leiden mutation. These patients require an aggressive strategy to prevent thromboembolism and to prevent excessive perioperative bleeding, for which they are increased risk as well. A hematology/vascular medicine consultation is recommended to help decide on an optimal antithrombotic plan that may include bridging. Mechanical compression devices and early mobilization are important postoperative measures to decrease the risk of VTE. Other strategies recommended include reducing vascular trauma by avoiding tourniquets and unnecessary blood draws and decreasing the number of blood pressure measurements to reduce cuff-induced stasis.[77]

URGENT REVERSAL OF ANTICOAGULATION

Rapid reversal of anticoagulation or antiplatelet therapy may occasionally be required, either preoperatively for emergency surgery or in the event of postoperative or traumatic bleeding. The antithrombotic agent and the urgency to return to normal coagulation profile determine the reversal strategy used in such instances.

VKA agents are commonly reversed with 24 to 48 hours by vitamin K in either oral or IV form. IV vitamin K has been associated with rare anaphylaxis and should be used judiciously.[78] Fresh frozen plasma (FFP) and PCCs are used for immediate reversal of VKA activity. PCCs rapidly reverse VKA-induced coagulopathy but are also low volume, thus may be a better option than FFP in patients in whom large volume transfusion cannot be tolerated (eg, patients with heart failure). The NOACs have no specific reversal agents and strategies suggested include the use of PCCs and dialysis for dabigatran; supportive measures, including whole blood or component transfusions, should also be considered.

At least 50% of functional platelets is required for hemostasis.[57] Platelet transfusion may be used in cases of ASA and other nonreversible antiplatelet agents but may not be as effective if given within 16 hours of the last intake.[57]

SUMMARY

The perioperative management of antithrombotic therapy is best determined by assessing the balance between the risks of surgical bleeding and thromboembolism in each patient. Although guidelines are available to assist with decision making, management of antithrombotic medication should be individualized with input from multiple disciplines as well as the patient.

REFERENCES

1. O'Donnell M, Kearon C. Perioperative management of oral anticoagulation. Cardiol Clin 2008;26(2): 299–309, viii.
2. Bradbury A, Adam D, Garrioch M, et al. Changes in platelet count, coagulation and fibrinogen associated with elective repair of asymptomatic abdominal aortic aneurysm and aortic reconstruction for occlusive disease. Eur J Vasc Endovasc Surg 1997;13(4): 375–80.
3. Heit JA, Mohr DN, Silverstein MD, et al. Predictors of recurrence after deep vein thrombosis and pulmonary embolism: a population-based cohort study. Arch Intern Med 2000;160(6):761–8.
4. Heit JA, O'Fallon WM, Petterson TM, et al. Relative impact of risk factors for deep vein thrombosis and pulmonary embolism: a population-based study. Arch Intern Med 2002;162(11):1245–8.
5. Kearon C, Hirsh J. Management of anticoagulation before and after elective surgery. N Engl J Med 1997;336(21):1506–11.
6. Douketis JD, Spyropoulos AC, Spencer FA, et al. Perioperative management of antithrombotic therapy: antithrombotic therapy and prevention of thrombosis, 9th ed: American College of Chest Physicians evidence-based clinical practice guidelines. Chest 2012;141(2 Suppl):e326S–50S.
7. Eijgenraam P, ten Cate H, ten Cate-Hoek AJ. Practice of bridging anticoagulation: guideline adherence and risk factors for bleeding. Neth J Med 2014;72(3):157–64.
8. Omran H, Bauersachs R, Rubenacker S, et al. The HAS-BLED score predicts bleedings during bridging of chronic oral anticoagulation. Results from the national multicentre BNK Online bRiDging REgistRy (BORDER). Thromb Haemost 2012; 108(1):65–73.
9. Darvish-Kazem S, Gandhi M, Marcucci M, et al. Perioperative management of antiplatelet therapy in patients with a coronary stent who need noncardiac surgery: a systematic review of clinical practice guidelines. Chest 2013;144(6):1848–56.
10. Nishimura RA, Otto CM, Bonow RO, et al. 2014 AHA/ACC guideline for the management of patients with valvular heart disease: a report of the American College of Cardiology/American Heart Association Task Force on Practice Guidelines. Circulation 2014;129(23):e521–643.
11. Fleisher LA, Fleischmann KE, Auerbach AD, et al. 2014 ACC/AHA guideline on perioperative cardiovascular evaluation and management of patients undergoing noncardiac surgery: a report of the American College of Cardiology/American Heart Association Task Force on Practice Guidelines. J Am Coll Cardiol 2014;64(22):e77–137.
12. Wysokinski WE, McBane RD, Daniels PR, et al. Periprocedural anticoagulation management of patients with nonvalvular atrial fibrillation. Mayo Clin Proc 2008;83(6):639–45.
13. Douketis JD, Johnson JA, Turpie AG. Low-molecular-weight heparin as bridging anticoagulation during interruption of warfarin: assessment of a standardized periprocedural anticoagulation regimen. Arch Intern Med 2004;164(12):1319–26.
14. Heidbuchel H, Verhamme P, Alings M, et al. EHRA practical guide on the use of new oral anticoagulants in patients with non-valvular atrial fibrillation: executive summary. Eur Heart J 2013;34(27): 2094–106.
15. Eerenberg ES, Kamphuisen PW, Sijpkens MK, et al. Reversal of rivaroxaban and dabigatran by prothrombin complex concentrate: a randomized, placebo-controlled, crossover study in healthy subjects. Circulation 2011;124(14):1573–9.
16. Kitslaar DB, Wysokinski WE, McBane RD 2nd. The role of novel anticoagulants in the management of venous thromboembolic disease. Curr Treat Options Cardiovasc Med 2014;16(8):326.
17. Secondary prevention in non-rheumatic atrial fibrillation after transient ischaemic attack or minor stroke. EAFT (European Atrial Fibrillation Trial) Study Group. Lancet 1993;342(8882):1255–62.
18. Salem DN, Stein PD, Al-Ahmad A, et al. Antithrombotic therapy in valvular heart disease–native and prosthetic: the Seventh ACCP Conference on Antithrombotic and Thrombolytic Therapy. Chest 2004; 126(3 Suppl):457S–82S.
19. Dzeshka MS, Lip GY. Specific risk scores for specific purposes: use CHA2DS2-VASc for assessing stroke risk, and use HAS-BLED for assessing bleeding risk in atrial fibrillation. Thromb Res 2014; 134(2):217–8.
20. Kaatz S, Douketis JD, Zhou H, et al. Risk of stroke after surgery in patients with and without chronic atrial fibrillation. J Thromb Haemost 2010;8(5): 884–90.
21. Risk factors for stroke and efficacy of antithrombotic therapy in atrial fibrillation. Analysis of pooled data from five randomized controlled trials. Arch Intern Med 1994;154(13):1449–57.
22. Echocardiographic predictors of stroke in patients with atrial fibrillation: a prospective study of 1066

patients from 3 clinical trials. Arch Intern Med 1998;158(12):1316–20.
23. Hart RG, Halperin JL. Atrial fibrillation and thromboembolism: a decade of progress in stroke prevention. Ann Intern Med 1999;131(9):688–95.
24. Singer DE, Albers GW, Dalen JE, et al. Antithrombotic therapy in atrial fibrillation: the seventh ACCP conference on antithrombotic and thrombolytic therapy. Chest 2004;126(3 Suppl):429S–56S.
25. van Diepen S, Youngson E, Ezekowitz JA, et al. Which risk score best predicts perioperative outcomes in nonvalvular atrial fibrillation patients undergoing noncardiac surgery? Am Heart J 2014;168(1):60–7.e5.
26. Tosetto A, Iorio A, Marcucci M, et al. Predicting disease recurrence in patients with previous unprovoked venous thromboembolism: a proposed prediction score (DASH). J Thromb Haemost 2012;10(6):1019–25.
27. Agnelli G, Prandoni P, Santamaria MG, et al. Three months versus one year of oral anticoagulant therapy for idiopathic deep venous thrombosis. Warfarin Optimal Duration Italian Trial Investigators. N Engl J Med 2001;345(3):165–9.
28. Tafur AJ, Wysokinski WE, McBane RD, et al. Cancer effect on periprocedural thromboembolism and bleeding in anticoagulated patients. Ann Oncol 2012;23(8):1998–2005.
29. Coon WW, Willis PW 3rd. Recurrence of venous thromboembolism. Surgery 1973;73(6):823–7.
30. Dunn AS, Turpie AG. Perioperative management of patients receiving oral anticoagulants: a systematic review. Arch Intern Med 2003;163(8):901–8.
31. White RH. ACP Journal Club. Scores poorly predict major bleeding (c-statistics </= 0.61) during oral anticoagulant therapy. Ann Intern Med 2013;158(6):JC13.
32. Gulec S. Misinterpretation of the HAS-BLED bleeding score by end-users. Thromb Res 2014;134(1):203.
33. Pisters R, Lane DA, Nieuwlaat R, et al. A novel user-friendly score (HAS-BLED) to assess 1-year risk of major bleeding in patients with atrial fibrillation: the Euro Heart Survey. Chest 2010;138(5):1093–100.
34. Chee YL, Crawford JC, Watson HG, et al. Guidelines on the assessment of bleeding risk prior to surgery or invasive procedures. British Committee for Standards in Haematology. Br J Haematol 2008;140(5):496–504.
35. McBane RD, Wysokinski WE, Daniels PR, et al. Periprocedural anticoagulation management of patients with venous thromboembolism. Arterioscler Thromb Vasc Biol 2010;30(3):442–8.
36. Pengo V, Cucchini U, Denas G, et al. Standardized low-molecular-weight heparin bridging regimen in outpatients on oral anticoagulants undergoing invasive procedure or surgery: an inception cohort management study. Circulation 2009;119(22):2920–7.
37. Lee AY, Rickles FR, Julian JA, et al. Randomized comparison of low molecular weight heparin and coumarin derivatives on the survival of patients with cancer and venous thromboembolism. J Clin Oncol 2005;23(10):2123–9.
38. Berge E, Abdelnoor M, Nakstad PH, et al. Low molecular-weight heparin versus aspirin in patients with acute ischaemic stroke and atrial fibrillation: a double-blind randomised study. HAEST Study Group. Heparin in Acute Embolic Stroke Trial. Lancet 2000;355(9211):1205–10.
39. Hart RG, Palacio S, Pearce LA. Atrial fibrillation, stroke, and acute antithrombotic therapy: analysis of randomized clinical trials. Stroke 2002;33(11):2722–7.
40. Saxena R, Lewis S, Berge E, et al. Risk of early death and recurrent stroke and effect of heparin in 3169 patients with acute ischemic stroke and atrial fibrillation in the International Stroke Trial. Stroke 2001;32(10):2333–7.
41. White RH, McKittrick T, Hutchinson R, et al. Temporary discontinuation of warfarin therapy: changes in the international normalized ratio. Ann Intern Med 1995;122(1):40–2.
42. Hylek EM, Regan S, Go AS, et al. Clinical predictors of prolonged delay in return of the international normalized ratio to within the therapeutic range after excessive anticoagulation with warfarin. Ann Intern Med 2001;135(6):393–400.
43. O'Donnell M, Kearon C. Perioperative management of oral anticoagulation. Clin Geriatr Med 2006;22(1):199–213, xi.
44. Sie P, Samama CM, Godier A, et al. Surgery and invasive procedures in patients on long-term treatment with direct oral anticoagulants: thrombin or factor-Xa inhibitors. Recommendations of the working group on perioperative haemostasis and the French Study Group on Thrombosis and Haemostasis. Arch Cardiovasc Dis 2011;104(12):669–76.
45. O'Donnell MJ, Kearon C, Johnson J, et al. Brief communication: Preoperative anticoagulant activity after bridging low-molecular-weight heparin for temporary interruption of warfarin. Ann Intern Med 2007;146(3):184–7.
46. Dunn AS, Spyropoulos AC, Turpie AG. Bridging therapy in patients on long-term oral anticoagulants who require surgery: the prospective peri-operative enoxaparin cohort trial (PROSPECT). J Thromb Haemost 2007;5(11):2211–8.
47. Eberli D, Chassot PG, Sulser T, et al. Urological surgery and antiplatelet drugs after cardiac and cerebrovascular accidents. J Urol 2010;183(6):2128–36.
48. van Kuijk JP, Flu WJ, Schouten O, et al. Timing of noncardiac surgery after coronary artery stenting

with bare metal or drug-eluting stents. Am J Cardiol 2009;104(9):1229–34.
49. Yusuf S, Zhao F, Mehta SR, et al. Effects of clopidogrel in addition to aspirin in patients with acute coronary syndromes without ST-segment elevation. N Engl J Med 2001;345(7):494–502.
50. Wiviott SD, Braunwald E, McCabe CH, et al. Prasugrel versus clopidogrel in patients with acute coronary syndromes. N Engl J Med 2007;357(20): 2001–15.
51. Gandhi NK, Abdel-Karim AR, Banerjee S, et al. Frequency and risk of noncardiac surgery after drug-eluting stent implantation. Catheter Cardiovasc Interv 2011;77(7):972–6.
52. Huang PH, Croce KJ, Bhatt DL, et al. Recommendations for management of antiplatelet therapy in patients undergoing elective noncardiac surgery after coronary stent implantation. Crit Pathw Cardiol 2012;11(4):177–85.
53. Wijeysundera DN, Wijeysundera HC, Yun L, et al. Risk of elective major noncardiac surgery after coronary stent insertion: a population-based study. Circulation 2012;126(11):1355–62.
54. Artang R, Dieter RS. Analysis of 36 reported cases of late thrombosis in drug-eluting stents placed in coronary arteries. Am J Cardiol 2007; 99(8):1039–43.
55. Grines CL, Bonow RO, Casey DE Jr, et al. Prevention of premature discontinuation of dual antiplatelet therapy in patients with coronary artery stents: a science advisory from the American Heart Association, American College of Cardiology, society for cardiovascular angiography and interventions, American College of Surgeons, and American Dental Association, with representation from the American College of Physicians. Circulation 2007;115(6):813–8.
56. Holmes DR Jr, Kereiakes DJ, Garg S, et al. Stent thrombosis. J Am Coll Cardiol 2010;56(17):1357–65.
57. Abualsaud AO, Eisenberg MJ. Perioperative management of patients with drug-eluting stents. JACC Cardiovasc Interv 2010;3(2):131–42.
58. Schwartz RS, Chronos NA, Virmani R. Preclinical restenosis models and drug-eluting stents: still important, still much to learn. J Am Coll Cardiol 2004;44(7):1373–85.
59. Awata M, Kotani J, Uematsu M, et al. Serial angioscopic evidence of incomplete neointimal coverage after sirolimus-eluting stent implantation: comparison with bare-metal stents. Circulation 2007; 116(8):910–6.
60. Sanon S, Rihal CS. Non-cardiac surgery after percutaneous coronary intervention. Am J Cardiol 2014; 114(10):1613–20.
61. Otsuka F, Vorpahl M, Nakano M, et al. Pathology of second-generation everolimus-eluting stents versus first-generation sirolimus- and paclitaxel-eluting stents in humans. Circulation 2014;129(2):211–23.
62. Albaladejo P, Marret E, Piriou V, et al. Perioperative management of antiplatelet agents in patients with coronary stents: recommendations of a French Task Force. Br J Anaesth 2006;97(4):580–2.
63. Cruden NL, Harding SA, Flapan AD, et al. Previous coronary stent implantation and cardiac events in patients undergoing noncardiac surgery. Circ Cardiovasc Interv 2010;3(3):236–42.
64. Schouten O, Bax JJ, Damen J, et al. Coronary artery stent placement immediately before noncardiac surgery: a potential risk? Anesthesiology 2007;106(5): 1067–9.
65. Reddy PR, Vaitkus PT. Risks of noncardiac surgery after coronary stenting. Am J Cardiol 2005;95(6): 755–7.
66. Oscarsson A, Gupta A, Fredrikson M, et al. To continue or discontinue aspirin in the perioperative period: a randomized, controlled clinical trial. Br J Anaesth 2010;104(3):305–12.
67. Burger W, Chemnitius JM, Kneissl GD, et al. Low-dose aspirin for secondary cardiovascular prevention - cardiovascular risks after its perioperative withdrawal versus bleeding risks with its continuation - review and meta-analysis. J Intern Med 2005; 257(5):399–414.
68. Ben Morrison T, Horst BM, Brown MJ, et al. Bridging with glycoprotein IIb/IIIa inhibitors for periprocedural management of antiplatelet therapy in patients with drug eluting stents. Catheter Cardiovasc Interv 2012;79(4):575–82.
69. Alshawabkeh LI, Prasad A, Lenkovsky F, et al. Outcomes of a preoperative " bridging" strategy with glycoprotein IIb/IIIa inhibitors to prevent perioperative stent thrombosis in patients with drug-eluting stents who undergo surgery necessitating interruption of thienopyridine administration. EuroIntervention 2013;9(2):204–11.
70. Kearon C, Akl EA, Comerota AJ, et al. Antithrombotic therapy for VTE disease: antithrombotic therapy and prevention of thrombosis, 9th ed: American College of Chest Physicians evidence-based clinical practice guidelines. Chest 2012;141(2 Suppl): e419S–94S.
71. Baglin TP, Brush J, Streiff M. Guidelines on use of vena cava filters. Br J Haematol 2006;134(6): 590–5.
72. Rajasekhar A, Streiff MB. Vena cava filters for management of venous thromboembolism: a clinical review. Blood Rev 2013;27(5):225–41.
73. Decousus H, Leizorovicz A, Parent F, et al. A clinical trial of vena caval filters in the prevention of pulmonary embolism in patients with proximal deep-vein thrombosis. Prevention du Risque d'Embolie Pulmonaire par Interruption Cave Study Group. N Engl J Med 1998;338(7):409–15.
74. Streiff MB. Vena caval filters: a comprehensive review. Blood 2000;95(12):3669–77.

75. Szucs G, Ajzner E, Muszbek L, et al. Assessment of thrombotic risk factors predisposing to thromboembolic complications in prosthetic orthopedic surgery. J Orthop Sci 2009;14(5):484–90.
76. Marchiori A, Mosena L, Prins MH, et al. The risk of recurrent venous thromboembolism among heterozygous carriers of factor V Leiden or prothrombin G20210A mutation. A systematic review of prospective studies. Haematologica 2007;92(8):1107–14.
77. Saunders KH, Erkan D, Lockshin MD. Perioperative management of antiphospholipid antibody-positive patients. Curr Rheumatol Rep 2014;16(7):426.
78. Fiore LD, Scola MA, Cantillon CE, et al. Anaphylactoid reactions to vitamin K. J Thromb Thrombolysis 2001;11(2):175–83.

Cardiopulmonary Bypass and Extracorporeal Life Support for Emergent Intraoperative Thoracic Situations

Tiago N. Machuca, MD, Marcelo Cypel, MD, Shaf Keshavjee, MD*

KEYWORDS

• Cardiopulmonary bypass • Extracorporeal life support • Extracorporeal membrane oxygenation • Lung cancer • Lung transplantation

KEY POINTS

- Initiation of extracorporeal life support during intraoperative thoracic surgical catastrophes can be lifesaving.
- Detailed knowledge of the different modes of support available can aid surgeons in decision making for identifying the ideal mode required for each scenario.
- Clear communication and effective team coordination are crucial.

INTRODUCTION

The availability of cardiopulmonary bypass (CPB) or extracorporeal life support (ECLS) (also referred to as extracorporeal membrane oxygenation [ECMO]) to support a patient during an intraoperative thoracic surgical crisis can be lifesaving. Common causes of intraoperative cardiac arrest, such as hemorrhagic shock and hypoxia, can be managed with either CPB or ECMO, depending on the degree of support required for different levels of complexity. With increasing applications of ECLS in thoracic surgery (such as in bridge to lung transplant, intraoperative lung transplant support, and bridge to recovery after lung transplantation), being knowledgeable about the capabilities and differences between CPB, venoarterial (VA) ECMO, and venovenous (VV) ECMO can guide rapid intraoperative decisions under stressful conditions and greatly benefit patients (**Fig. 1**).

After a brief review of predictors of intraoperative mortality in noncardiac surgery, this article addresses potential applications and the reported clinical experience with CPB, VA-ECMO, and VV-ECMO in thoracic surgical procedures.

PREDICTORS OF OPERATIVE MORTALITY AND AVOIDABLE FACTORS

Intraoperative cardiac arrest poses a unique situation. The patient is fully monitored and the medical team is readily available to react to the causative factor. In the past, intraoperative cardiac arrest was divided into anesthesia related, surgery related, or related to patient characteristics and reason for surgery.[1] Among the anesthesia-related causes, airway issues and medication

Disclosure: The authors have nothing to disclose.
Division of Thoracic Surgery, Toronto General Hospital, University Health Network, University of Toronto, 200 Elizabeth Street, 9N-946, Toronto, Ontario M5G 2C4, Canada
* Corresponding author. Toronto General Hospital, 200 Elizabeth Street, 9N-946, Toronto, Ontario M5G 2C4, Canada.
E-mail address: shaf.keshavjee@uhn.ca

Thorac Surg Clin 25 (2015) 325–334
http://dx.doi.org/10.1016/j.thorsurg.2015.04.012
1547-4127/15/$ – see front matter

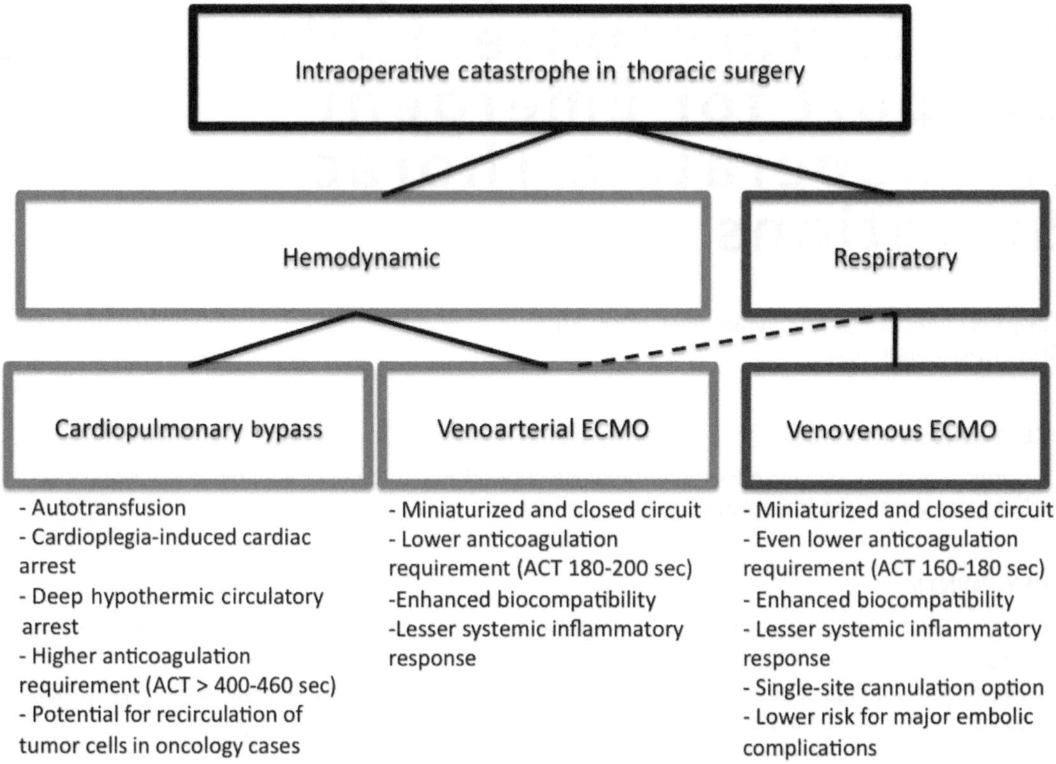

Fig. 1. Features of different modes of support for thoracic surgery intraoperative catastrophes. ACT, activated clotting time.

side effects are commonly associated with arrest. Among the surgical factors, bleeding is often highlighted. In a large study comprising 518,294 patients, with 223 intraoperative arrests, factor such as high American Society of Anesthesiologists (ASA) score, general anesthesia, emergent procedures, use of vasopressors before arrest, protracted hypotension before arrest, bleeding as the cause of arrest, and arrest during nonstandard working hours were all associated with worse survival after resuscitative measures.[2] However, on a multivariate analysis, only bleeding, documented hypotension, nonstandard working hours, and diabetes proved to be independent predictors of survival. Although 34.5% of patients experiencing intraoperative arrest survived to hospital discharge, these numbers decreased to 10.3% when the arrest was attributed to bleeding.

In a more recent multicenter study from the American College of Surgeons National Surgical Quality Improvement Program database (362,767 patients; 0.072% intraoperative arrest with a 62% 30-day mortality), Goswami and colleagues[3] showed that, among factors such as emergent surgery, ASA score, and preoperative comorbidities, intraoperative blood transfusion was the most striking factor associated with intraoperative cardiac arrest. More importantly, there was a dose-dependent correlation with intraoperative arrest, with adjusted odds ratios of 2.5 (95% confidence interval [CI], 1.69–3.71), 7.59 (95% CI, 4.94–11.67), 11.4 (95% CI, 6.22–20.88), and 29.68 (95% CI, 18.66–47.18) if the patient required 1 to 3, 4 to 6, 7 to 9, or greater than or equal to 10 units of packed red blood cells, respectively.

Focusing on patients who experienced intraoperative cardiac arrest but were successfully resuscitated and made it to intensive care unit (ICU) recovery (total 140, with 20.7% thoracic surgery patients), Constant and colleagues[1] showed a 45.7% ICU mortality, mostly caused by multiple organ failure. In contrast, 45.3% of patients were alive at 90-day follow-up with either good cerebral function or enough function to perform daily activities. Independent predictors of favorable neurologic outcome were ventricular fibrillation/tachycardia as the first recorded rhythm and no use of epinephrine to treat postarrest shock (reflecting the severity of shock). A similar large multicenter study has also reinforced the correlation of ventricular fibrillation/tachycardia as the primary arrest rhythm and improved outcomes.[4]

USE OF CARDIOPULMONARY BYPASS IN THORACIC SURGERY

Emergent Use of Cardiopulmonary Bypass in Thoracic Surgery

Use of CPB can be lifesaving in emergent scenarios such as massive uncontrollable bleeding or respiratory instability. Whenever possible, especially in extended resections, it is important to anticipate the potential need for CPB. Thoughtful anticipatory patient positioning and prepping can be helpful in emergent situations. For example, in lateral or posterolateral thoracotomies, including the ipsilateral groin in the prepped surgical field and even inserting femoral arterial and venous catheters can avoid the need for emergent percutaneous vessel puncture or cutdown dissection in hypotensive patients.

Personnel are crucial in stressful, potentially fatal scenarios. Having an available perfusionist as well as a primed pump on standby for potential CPB is ideal. Moreover, an experienced anesthetist or even a second one is invaluable in catastrophic scenarios. Scrub and circulating nurses familiar with procedures on CPB should join the team if not already in the room. If operating with a trainee, the surgeon should consider having a second attending surgeon scrub. In addition, it is common for a room with an ongoing intraoperative catastrophe to become crowded and noisy. Having several voices talking at the same time is not productive. Leadership from the surgical and anesthesia sides should work in a close relationship to run the code. Communication should be clear and the whole team should be made aware of the current intraoperative catastrophe and the specific management plan.

The surgeon should be diligent and recognize that unsuccessful attempts to correct a life-threatening hemorrhage under suboptimal conditions will only make things worse. A sponge stick, clamps, or the hand should be used to control the source of bleeding while the required resources become available, including blood in the room and, ideally, activation of a massive transfusion protocol.

Exposure is key to allowing adequate patient cannulation and repair of the injured structure. In cases of video-assisted or robot-assisted procedures, enlarging or creating a working incision is required. Surgeons should not hesitate to add an incision to achieve adequate exposure for CPB. In cases of anterior thoracotomy (such as in a left single-lung transplant), extension to transverse transection of the sternum is helpful, such as in a clamshell incision. Another incision that confers excellent mediastinal as well as ipsilateral pleural cavity exposure is the hemiclamshell incision. It may be used for resection of central tumors and offers central cannulation possibilities regardless of the side.

Cannulation options depending on different incisions are listed in **Table 1**. Similar steps to perform an adequate planned arterial cannulation, such as palpation of the aorta to avoid calcifications as well as correct cannula positioning to avoid intimal tear

Table 1
Cannulation strategies for either CPB or ECMO according to different incisions

Incision	Arterial	Venous
Right thoracotomy	Ascending aorta Femoral artery Axillary artery	Right atrium Femoral vein Axillary vein
Left thoracotomy	Descending aorta Ascending aorta Femoral artery Axillary artery	Femoral vein Pulmonary artery Right atrium Axillary vein
Clamshell	Ascending aorta Femoral artery Axillary artery	Right atrium Femoral vein Axillary vein
Right hemiclamshell	Ascending aorta Femoral artery Axillary artery	Right atrium Femoral vein Axillary vein
Left hemiclamshell	Descending aorta Ascending aorta Femoral artery Axillary artery	Right atrium Femoral vein Axillary vein

or cerebral overflow through the innominate artery, should be kept in mind during the emergent cannulation.

If the patient develops life-threatening instability and a decision is made to establish cardiopulmonary support, a bolus of heparin is given while appropriate access and exposure for cannulation is achieved. Note that the target activated clotting time (ACT) for CPB is usually more than 400 seconds, and for ECLS it is 180 to 200 seconds. This is an important decision juncture to consider if there is sufficient time depending on the operation being undertaken and the risk of operative field bleeding and coagulopathy. Appropriate temperature probes to monitor core temperature should be placed if not already done.

The surgeon should adapt the degree of support required to the intraoperative scenario. Note that most thoracic surgical crises can be managed with partial CPB. Nevertheless, total CPB with cardioplegic arrest, fibrillatory cardiac arrest, or deep hypothermic circulatory arrest may be used in more complex repairs. Furthermore, the use of mild to moderate hypothermia for end-organ protection should be considered, especially in cases with profound hypotension or cardiac arrest before institution of CPB.

The use of high-realism simulation coupled with principles of crew resource management has been shown to be effective in improving teamwork performance during critical scenarios.[5] One of the crisis management cases in this study was the initiation and management of CPB in a patient experiencing massive bleeding and hemodynamic instability during a mediastinal tumor resection. Debriefing sessions using videos of the event were performed after each scenario in order to discuss both individual and team performances. Significant positive changes in behavior were observed and most participants recommended periodic repeat simulation educational sessions. An adaptation of crew resource management in a thoracic surgical crisis managed with CPB/ECMO is shown in **Box 1**.

Another area of recent focus is the use of crisis checklists to improve patient safety and team performance in the operating room. Ziewacz and colleagues[6] identified the most frequent operating room crises (such as cardiac arrest, failed airway, hemorrhage, hypotension, and hypoxia) and their corresponding metrics of essential care. In a pilot simulation including 2 teams, the team using a checklist presented a 4% rate of failure to adhere to critical steps, whereas the team working from memory alone presented a 24% failure rate. In a validation of this previous study, done with 17 operating room teams, use of the checklist resulted in a 6% failure rate versus a 23% failure rate in the scenarios without it.[7] In the end, 97% of study participants reportedly wanted a checklist available for the operating team if any of the crisis scenarios were to happen with them as patients. In contrast with the universally used World Health Organization checklist for safe surgery, which focuses on aspects such as the correct operation on the correct patient on the correct side, safe anesthesia, and minimizing infectious complications, the crisis checklist is only activated when dealing with a catastrophic intraoperative scenario.[8] It comprises a color-coded algorithm-based approach for each of the 12 most frequently seen crisis, guiding the team through diagnosis of potential causative sources as well as the most appropriate management plan.

Outcomes of Cardiopulmonary Bypass with Resection of Thoracic Malignancies

Although uncommonly used, CPB may be an important adjunct to allow for curative intent resection of advanced lung cancer and other thoracic malignancies (**Fig. 2**). Nevertheless, theoretic considerations, such as pump-related immunosuppression or vascular tumor dissemination, should be weighed on an individual basis during surgical planning.[9,10]

In one of the largest studies to date, Byrne and colleagues[9] described 8 patients who underwent planned CPB (4 lesions invading pulmonary artery, 3 left atrium, and 1 superior vena cava) and 6 patients who required emergent CPB to correct great vessel injury (2 superior vena cava, 2 inferior vena cava, and 2 pulmonary artery). One patient died on the first postoperative day because of tumor embolus (metastatic chondrosarcoma with planned palliative resection). Complications related to CPB included low cardiac output syndrome, postoperative bleeding requiring reoperation, stroke, and pulmonary edema. In the emergent CPB group, mild to moderate hypothermia was used, with a mean temperature of 30 ± 6°C. With follow-up ranging from 2 to 107 months, 1-year and 3-year survivals were 57% and 36%, respectively.

Hasegawa and colleagues[11] reported on 11 patients with a median age of 62 years who underwent extended lung resections on CPB. The investigators considered for surgical procedure patients with cT4N0-1M0 (7 patients) or single-level N2 (4 patients). Indications for CPB included resection of pulmonary artery trunk, aorta, and left atrium. The 30-day mortality was zero and 1 patient had hospital mortality caused by mediastinitis. Eight patients died because of recurrence

Box 1
Crew resource management principles in emergent CPB/ECLS

1. Clarify roles
    a. Explicitly establish the event manager (team leader)
        i. Step back and manage the event
        ii. Articulate clear goal to the team (inform about the ongoing catastrophe and management plan)
        iii. Organize the team (anesthesia, perfusion, nursing)
        iv. Control communication (voice of command)
    b. Participants explicitly assume a responsibility
    c. Stay aware of the whole situation
    d. Help with event management
2. Communicate effectively
    a. Address people directly
    b. Close the loop
3. Use support well
    a. Call for help early (blood bank, extra surgeon, extra anesthesiologist, pump-familiar operating room nurse, perfusionist)
    b. Orient your helpers to the issue, the action, and the background (clearly inform modifications in incision and proposed cannulation strategy)
    c. Consider taking people out of their traditional jobs
4. Avoid fixation
    a. Step back
    b. Verbalize, review frequently (do not forget heparin)
    c. Invite input, open possibilities (debriefing after resolution)
5. Manage resources
    a. Plan ahead (anticipation, catheters in place, pump room, perfusionist on standby)
    b. Understand the infrastructure
    c. Think "out of the box" (what is the ideal mode of support to manage this scenario?)

Adapted from Stevens LM, Cooper JB, Raemer DB, et al. Educational program in crisis management for cardiac surgery teams including high realism simulation. J Thorac Cardiovasc Surg 2012;144:17–24.

after a median of 254 days, whereas 2 patients were alive but with local recurrent disease.

Another Japanese series described 16 patients who underwent lung resection concomitant with thoracic aorta resection.[12] CPB was required in 10 patients, whereas a passive ascending-to-descending aorta shunt was used in 4 patients. Although 5 patients died because of recurrence, 9 were alive after a median follow-up of 54 months. Nodal status was an important prognostic factor, with a 5-year survival going from 70% to 17% for patients with N0 versus N2 to N3 disease, respectively. Although this study suggests that favorable outcomes can be achieved with this strategy, recent reports have described the successful use of aortic endografting to facilitate the resection of malignancies invading the aorta.[13] In the series of Collaud and colleagues,[14] 3 patients with involvement of the descending aorta and 2 with involvement of the aortic arch were treated with such a strategy. CPB was avoided in all cases and the 5 patients were alive after a median follow-up of 39 months.

In the report of de Perrot and colleagues,[15] 5 patients required CPB for great vessel resection, whereas in 2 cases CPB was initiated during carinal resection. All patients were successfully discharged home. However, both patients undergoing carinal resection required unplanned CPB because of pulmonary edema on the lung

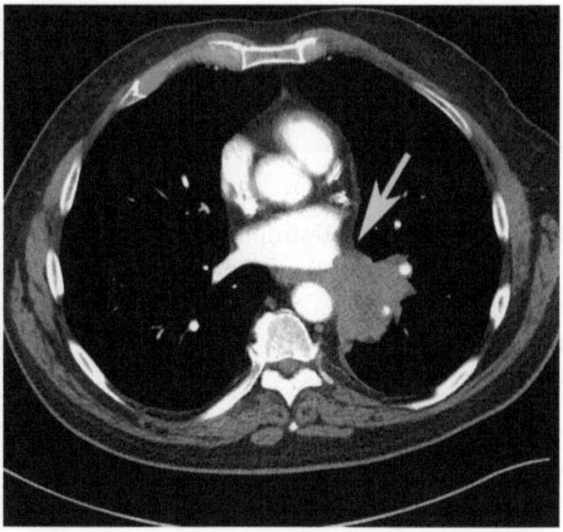

Fig. 2. Patient with a cT4N0M0 lung cancer, with potential invasion of the aorta and left atrium. Resection was planned with cardiopulmonary support on standby. After careful operative inspection, although there was no invasion of the descending aorta, direct extension into the left atrium was found. CPB with cardioplegic arrest was used to allow safe and wide opening of the left atrium with subsequent reconstruction. (*Arrow* indicates area of left atrial invasion).

being ventilated and had a protracted postoperative course, with pneumonia (discharged at postoperative day 25) and acute respiratory distress syndrome (discharged at postoperative day 91). One patient died after 6 months and 6 patients were alive with follow-up ranging from 8 to 72 months.

Muralidaran and colleagues[16] performed a systematic review of 20 articles reporting on outcomes of CPB use for resection of primary lung cancer. With a total of 72 patients (mean age, 55 $\pm$ 10 years), most patients had stage IIIB cancer (84%, but most likely using the previous International Association for the Study of Lung Cancer staging system with T4N0 being stage IIIB) and underwent a pneumonectomy (74%). The adjacent organs resected were most often aorta (43%), left atrium (25%), and pulmonary artery (11%). The 5-year survival was 37%. On both univariate and multivariate analysis, the use of planned versus emergent CPB was the only significant factor associated with survival (hazard ratio, 0.28; 95% CI, 0.09–0.90) (**Fig. 3**). Operative mortality was virtually zero in this review, which strongly suggests a general reporting bias. Nevertheless, the investigators highlight that these findings reinforce the concept that favorable outcomes can be achieved in a highly selected population.

Contrary to these previous reports, the study from the Memorial Sloan-Kettering Cancer Center excluded patients with bronchogenic carcinoma, with a final cohort of 10 patients with mainly soft tissue sarcomas invading the great vessels and/or heart.[17] Seven patients required planned CPB. There were no operative mortalities. The median requirement for packed red blood cells transfusion was 6 units and 1 patient required reoperation

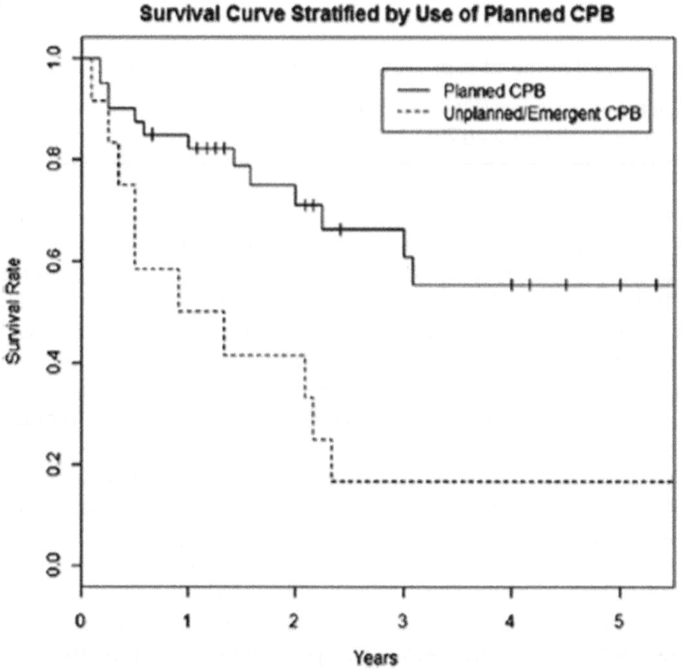

Fig. 3. Survival according to the use of planned versus unplanned CPB for primary lung cancer. The data are from a systematic review of 20 articles including 71 patients. (*From* Muralidaran A, Detterbeck FC, Boffa DJ, et al. Long-term survival after lung resection for non-small cell lung cancer with circulatory bypass: a systematic review. J Thorac Cardiovasc Surg 2011;142:1137–42; with permission.)

because of bleeding. One important aspect that should be highlighted in this study is that although R0 resection was performed in only 1 case, patients in this series were highly symptomatic (massive hemoptysis, superior vena cava syndrome, bilateral pulmonary embolism, and distal arterial embolization) and often an R2 palliative resection was planned. The median postoperative hospital stay was 6 days, reflecting the low morbidity in this series. Patients with R0 and R1 resections experienced median survivals of 21.7 and 33.3 months, respectively.

Similarly, the report of Vaporciyan and colleagues, from the MD Anderson Cancer Center, included mostly metastatic lesions in symptomatic patients. The use of CPB (5 cases), CPB with cardiac arrest (12 cases), and CPB with deep hypothermic circulatory arrest (2 cases) shows how the surgical team can tailor different degrees of support according to the intraoperative scenario. The complete resection rate was 91% for the 11 patients whose operation had a curative intent. With a median follow-up of 27 months, the 1-year and 2-year survivals were 65% and 45%, respectively.

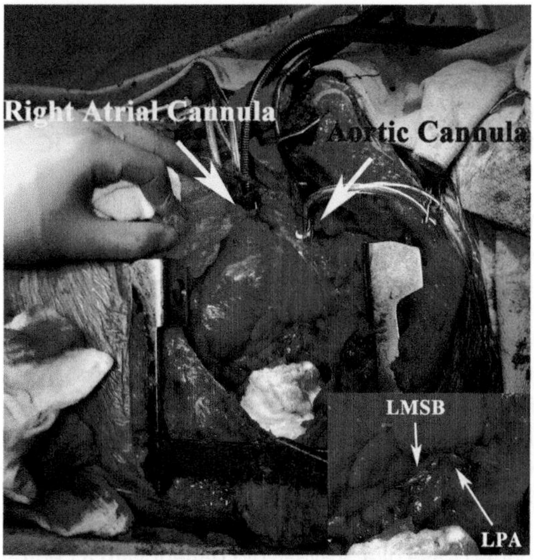

Fig. 4. A clamshell incision with a left postpneumonectomy space. The patient has a locally advanced thymoma invading the main left pulmonary artery. VA-ECMO was used through central cannulation in order to avoid hemodynamic instability during cardiac manipulation and unload the pulmonary circulation. LMSB, left mainstem bronchus; LPA, left pulmonary artery.

USE OF VENOARTERIAL EXTRACORPOREAL MEMBRANE OXYGENATION IN THORACIC SURGICAL PROCEDURES

ECMO has several theoretic advantages compared with CPB: (1) a miniaturized circuit that requires lower priming volumes; (2) a closed circulation circuit with no cardiotomy suction, limiting air-blood contact; and (3) enhanced biocompatibility leading to lesser anticoagulation requirement and potentially to lesser coagulopathy/systemic inflammatory response (**Fig. 4**). In a meta-analysis including 24 randomized studies of coronary artery bypass or aortic valve replacement, miniaturized biocompatible circuits led to lower risk of blood transfusion requirement (17.5% vs 43.1%), lesser neurologic events (2.3% vs 4%), lesser inotropic support, and lesser systemic inflammation, reflected in a shorter mechanical ventilation period, a shorter ICU stay, and more importantly lower hospital mortality (0.5% vs 1.7%).[18] Nevertheless, in cases of massive bleeding with difficult control, CPB provides the advantages of autotransfusion; rapid heterologous blood transfusion; delivery of cardioplegia for cardiac arrest; and, if needed, deep hypothermic circulatory arrest.

As described by Lang and colleagues,[10] VA-ECMO can be considered as an alternative to CPB in cases of complex resection of intrathoracic malignancies whenever there is no evidence of cardiac (requirement to open a heart chamber), aortic arch, or pulmonary trunk extension. In their series of 9 patients (6 for tracheobronchial resections and 3 because of great vessel infiltration), 8 patients left the hospital after a median of 10 days. No reoperation for bleeding was required, the median ICU stay was only 1 day, and the 1-year and 3-year survivals were both 76.7%. The investigators highlighted potential benefits of VA-ECMO compared with CPB for oncologic purposes, namely (1) less anticoagulation requirement in a patient who is likely to require extensive dissection; (2) a closed-circulation circuit, avoiding recirculation of tumor cells, debris, and cytokines that might be spilled into the surgical field; and (3) more biocompatibility, causing less systemic inflammation with less immunosuppression.

Kodama and colleagues[19] performed intrathoracic resections in 15 patients with VA-ECMO on standby. The support was required for 6 cases, with 1 emergent case of bleeding into the airway during resection of an esophageal cancer invading the membranous trachea. In this case VA-ECMO support was used for 6 hours to allow completion of the esophageal resection and tracheal reconstruction, which highlights the possibility of maintaining VA-ECMO support for longer periods without causing pump-related complications such as hemolysis, coagulopathy, and enhanced systemic inflammatory response syndrome.

USE OF VENOVENOUS EXTRACORPOREAL MEMBRANE OXYGENATION IN THORACIC SURGICAL PROCEDURES

With increasing technological improvements and cannulation advantages leading to less anticoagulation requirement and fewer complications than VA support,[20] VV-ECMO may be considered for support in cases of intraoperative emergent life-threatening respiratory instability, such as airway loss, pulmonary edema, and massive hemoptysis. Previously reported cases of CPB for tracheal or carinal resection in the early 2000s could benefit from this mode of support nowadays.[15,21]

This scenario is well illustrated by a recently reported case of a 36-year-old patient with a central airway squamous cell carcinoma obstructing the right and left mainstem bronchi while receiving definitive chemoradiation.[22] Hypoxic respiratory arrest occurred during line placement for an emergent rigid bronchoscopy and inadequate oxygenation was observed despite best efforts with standard rigid bronchoscopic debridement and endotracheal intubation. A dual-lumen single jugular cannula was then placed to support oxygenation to facilitate further rigid bronchoscopy for tumor debridement and placement of a Y-stent. The patient was weaned off ECLS, decannulated at the end of the procedure, and discharged home several days later with intact neurologic function.

Additional situations in which VV-ECMO has proved invaluable include the intraoperative management of previous pneumonectomy patients undergoing another thoracic procedure and in cases of massive pulmonary hemorrhage in patients with chronic thromboembolic pulmonary hypertension undergoing pulmonary thromboendarterectomy.[23,24] In this last scenario, support can be instituted without the need for anticoagulation, although care is necessary to maintain higher flows and the use of heparin-bonded circuits.[24]

LUNG TRANSPLANTATION: CARDIOPULMONARY BYPASS OR EXTRACORPOREAL MEMBRANE OXYGENATION?

Because of the advantages listed earlier, ECMO has replaced CPB as the first option for intraoperative cardiorespiratory support for lung transplantation in our center and many large-volume lung transplant centers. In our experience, a matched analysis of semielective cases (exclusion of emergent cases of massive bleeding and those bridged with ECMO) including 33 VA-ECMOs and 66 CPBs, the former resulted in lesser intraoperative blood product transfusion requirement (mean 3 vs 6 U of packed red blood cells; 0 vs 4 U of fresh-frozen plasma; 0 vs 1 U of adult pooled platelets), lesser mechanical ventilation requirement (3 vs 7.5 days), shorter ICU stay (5 vs 9.5 days), and ultimately shorter hospital stay (19 vs 27 days).[25]

In the experience of Bermudez and colleagues[26] comparing 49 VA-ECMOs with 222 CPBs at the University of Pittsburgh, there was a higher requirement for reintubation, tracheostomy, and dialysis in the CPB group. The lack of significant differences in perioperative blood transfusion requirement and hospital length of stay may have been caused by the ECMO group including a sicker population, as reflected by the higher lung allocation scores (73.3 vs 52.9) and higher pretransplantation ECLS requirement (42.8% vs 7.2%).

Another report supporting the use of ECMO for lung transplantation came from Columbia University.[27] With 47 ECMOs versus 55 CPBs, the investigators observed higher transfusion requirements (fresh-frozen plasma, platelets, cryoprecipitate, and cell saver volume), higher requirements for reoperation because of bleeding (38.2% vs 14.9%), and higher incidence of primary graft dysfunction at 72 hours (76.4% vs 56.5%) for the CPB group. Nevertheless, there was no difference in survival curves.

The experience of the group from Hannover, Germany, with 46 consecutive ECMOs compared with 46 consecutive CPBs also supports the use of VA-ECMO for lung transplantation.[28] Their analysis showed higher transfusion requirement (packed red blood cells and platelets); higher requirement for dialysis (48% vs 13%); higher need for new postoperative extracorporeal life support (26% vs 4%); and, more importantly, higher hospital mortality (39% vs 13%) for the CPB group. The investigators categorized the need for intraoperative support as planned (pulmonary hypertension as transplant indication, already on ECMO as a bridge, suprasystemic pulmonary artery pressures, or concomitant cardiac surgery procedure) or unplanned. There were more planned ECMOs than CPBs (61% vs 28%). Moreover, unplanned cases could be either elective (hemodynamic or respiratory instability on test ipsilateral pulmonary artery clamping and single-lung ventilation) or nonelective (cardiorespiratory instability during the implantation steps). There were no differences in the rate of nonelective support initiation between groups (30% CPB vs 22% ECMO).

In the largest study to date, Aigner and colleagues[29] reported on the use of intraoperative ECMO for 130 patients at the Medical University of Vienna, Austria. Although comparisons were confounded by most of the 27 CPB cases having concomitant cardiac procedures performed, there was a trend to shorter ICU stay and a significantly shorter hospital stay in the ECMO group. The preference for central cannulation was highlighted after their initial experience with groin cannulations resulting in intraoperative venous drainage issues during heart manipulation along with cases of vascular complications and lymphatic fistulas.

Based on this recent literature, there is growing evidence to support the use of VA-ECMO rather than CPB for lung transplantation. Nevertheless, preference should be given to CPB in cases of massive bleeding with difficult control and requirement of cardioplegic cardiac arrest for complex atrial or pulmonary artery anastomosis.

SUMMARY

Intraoperative thoracic surgical catastrophes, such as massive hemorrhage and respiratory instability, can benefit from the availability of extracorporeal circulation modes to support the patient while the appropriate repair is made.

Teamwork is key and, given the evidence supporting better performance with the use of simulation and surgical-crisis checklists, their use should be encouraged. Anticipation is another important factor because the results of intrathoracic malignancy resection are clearly superior in the setting of planned cardiopulmonary support. In addition, familiarity with the different modes of support that are currently available can direct the decision-making process toward the best option to facilitate resolution of the intraoperative catastrophe with the least related morbidity.

REFERENCES

1. Constant AL, Montlahuc C, Grimaldi D, et al. Predictors of functional outcome after intraoperative cardiac arrest. Anesthesiology 2014;121:482–91.
2. Sprung J, Warner ME, Contreras MG, et al. Predictors of survival following cardiac arrest in patients undergoing noncardiac surgery: a study of 518,294 patients at a tertiary referral center. Anesthesiology 2003;99:259–69.
3. Goswami S, Brady JE, Jordan DA, et al. Intraoperative cardiac arrests in adults undergoing noncardiac surgery: incidence, risk factors, and survival outcome. Anesthesiology 2012;117:1018–26.
4. Ramachandran SK, Mhyre J, Kheterpal S, et al. Predictors of survival from perioperative cardiopulmonary arrests: a retrospective analysis of 2,524 events from the Get With The Guidelines-Resuscitation registry. Anesthesiology 2013;119:1322–39.
5. Stevens LM, Cooper JB, Raemer DB, et al. Educational program in crisis management for cardiac surgery teams including high realism simulation. J Thorac Cardiovasc Surg 2012;144:17–24.
6. Ziewacz JE, Arriaga AF, Bader AM, et al. Crisis checklists for the operating room: development and pilot testing. J Am Coll Surg 2011;213:212–7.e10.
7. Arriaga AF, Bader AM, Wong JM, et al. Simulation-based trial of surgical-crisis checklists. N Engl J Med 2013;368:246–53.
8. Haynes AB, Weiser TG, Berry WR, et al. A surgical safety checklist to reduce morbidity and mortality in a global population. N Engl J Med 2009;360:491–9.
9. Byrne JG, Leacche M, Agnihotri AK, et al. The use of cardiopulmonary bypass during resection of locally advanced thoracic malignancies: a 10-year two-center experience. Chest 2004;125:1581–6.
10. Lang G, Taghavi S, Aigner C, et al. Extracorporeal membrane oxygenation support for resection of locally advanced thoracic tumors. Ann Thorac Surg 2011;92:264–70.
11. Hasegawa S, Bando T, Isowa N, et al. The use of cardiopulmonary bypass during extended resection of non-small cell lung cancer. Interact Cardiovasc Thorac Surg 2003;2:676–9.
12. Ohta M, Hirabayasi H, Shiono H, et al. Surgical resection for lung cancer with infiltration of the thoracic aorta. J Thorac Cardiovasc Surg 2005;129:804–8.
13. Marulli G, Lepidi S, Frigatti P, et al. Thoracic aorta endograft as an adjunct to resection of a locally invasive tumor: a new indication to endograft. J Vasc Surg 2008;47:868–70.
14. Collaud S, Waddell TK, Yasufuku K, et al. Thoracic aortic endografting facilitates the resection of tumors infiltrating the aorta. J Thorac Cardiovasc Surg 2014;147:1178–82 [discussion: 1182].
15. de Perrot M, Fadel E, Mussot S, et al. Resection of locally advanced (T4) non-small cell lung cancer with cardiopulmonary bypass. Ann Thorac Surg 2005;79:1691–6 [discussion: 1697].
16. Muralidaran A, Detterbeck FC, Boffa DJ, et al. Long-term survival after lung resection for non-small cell lung cancer with circulatory bypass: a systematic review. J Thorac Cardiovasc Surg 2011;142:1137–42.
17. Park BJ, Bacchetta M, Bains MS, et al. Surgical management of thoracic malignancies invading the heart or great vessels. Ann Thorac Surg 2004;78:1024–30.
18. Anastasiadis K, Antonitsis P, Haidich AB, et al. Use of minimal extracorporeal circulation improves outcome after heart surgery; a systematic review

and meta-analysis of randomized controlled trials. Int J Cardiol 2013;164:158–69.
19. Kodama K, Higashiyama M, Yokouchi H, et al. Use of percutaneous cardiopulmonary support (PCPS) for extended surgery in patients with T4 tumor. Kyobu Geka 2000;53:721–5 [discussion: 725–8]. [in Japanese].
20. Cypel M, Keshavjee S. Extracorporeal life support as a bridge to lung transplantation. Clin Chest Med 2011;32:245–51.
21. Tyagi I, Goyal A, Syal R, et al. Emergency cardiopulmonary bypass for impassable airway. J Laryngol Otol 2006;120:687–90.
22. Cypel M. Use of single cannula venous-venous extracorporeal life support in the management of life-threatening airway obstruction. Ann Thorac Surg 2015;99(3):e63–5.
23. Collins NF, Ellard L, Licari E, et al. Veno-venous extracorporeal membrane oxygenation and apnoeic oxygenation for tracheo-oesophageal fistula repair in a previously pneumonectomised patient. Anaesth Intensive Care 2014;42:789–92.
24. Cronin B, Maus T, Pretorius V, et al. Case 13-2014: management of pulmonary hemorrhage after pulmonary endarterectomy with venovenous extracorporeal membrane oxygenation without systemic anticoagulation. J Cardiothorac Vasc Anesth 2014;28:1667–76.
25. Machuca TN, Collaud S, Mercier O, et al. Outcomes of intraoperative ECMO versus cardiopulmonary bypass for lung transplantation. J Thorac Cardiovasc Surg 2015;149(4):1152–7.
26. Bermudez CA, Shiose A, Esper SA, et al. Outcomes of intraoperative venoarterial extracorporeal membrane oxygenation versus cardiopulmonary bypass during lung transplantation. Ann Thorac Surg 2014;98:1936–43.
27. Biscotti M, Yang J, Sonett J, et al. Comparison of extracorporeal membrane oxygenation versus cardiopulmonary bypass for lung transplantation. J Thorac Cardiovasc Surg 2014;148:2410–6.
28. Ius F, Kuehn C, Tudorache I, et al. Lung transplantation on cardiopulmonary support: venoarterial extracorporeal membrane oxygenation outperformed cardiopulmonary bypass. J Thorac Cardiovasc Surg 2012;144:1510–6.
29. Aigner C, Wisser W, Taghavi S, et al. Institutional experience with extracorporeal membrane oxygenation in lung transplantation. Eur J Cardiothorac Surg 2007;31:468–73 [discussion: 473–4].

Management of Complications After Pneumonectomy

Shawn S. Groth, MD, MS*, Bryan M. Burt, MD,
David J. Sugarbaker, MD

KEYWORDS

• Pneumonectomy • Postoperative complications • Postoperative care

KEY POINTS

- Mortalities after pneumonectomy have steadily declined over the last 80 years but morbidity remains significant.
- Following pneumonectomy, patients have limited cardiopulmonary reserve and therefore live along a narrow margin of error.
- Appropriate patient selection and a proactive approach to perioperative management are essential to optimizing outcomes after pneumonectomy.
- When complications do occur, they must be aggressively treated to curtail their potential impact on the patient.

The patient's outcome correlates directly with the surgeon's attention to a myriad of minor details. This obsession of doing a lot of little things right is the foundation for good surgical results.

—Hiram C. Polk, MD

Indeed, meticulous attention to detail is paramount for optimizing outcomes after pneumonectomy. As compared with lesser pulmonary resections, most single- and multi-institution studies over the last 80 years indicate that pneumonectomy is associated with the highest morbidity and mortality rates.[1,2] Complication rates after pneumonectomy, however, have steadily decreased with time, likely because of improvements in patient selection, operative techniques, and perioperative care. In fact, one recent multicenter study of select patients who underwent resection for early-stage non-small cell lung cancer found no significant difference in mortality after pneumonectomy, as compared with lobectomy.[3]

Although most complications of pulmonary resection are not immediately life-threatening, they are associated with increased cost, increased length of hospital stay,[4] and lower 5-year cancer-specific survival rates.[5] As such, it is imperative that thoracic surgeons understand the cause and management of potential complications of a standard pneumonectomy and extrapleural pneumonectomy (EPP) to proactively minimize their risk of occurrence and to curtail their impact when they do occur.

PATIENT SELECTION

Most pneumonectomies are done on an elective basis. As such, it is essential that patients who

The authors have nothing to disclose.
Division of General Thoracic Surgery, Michael E. DeBakey Department of Surgery, Baylor College of Medicine, One Baylor Plaza, Houston, TX 77030, USA
* Corresponding author. Division of General Thoracic Surgery, Michael E. DeBakey Department of Surgery, Baylor College of Medicine, One Baylor Plaza, BCM 390, Houston, TX 77005.
E-mail address: Shawn.Groth@bcm.edu

Thorac Surg Clin 25 (2015) 335–348
http://dx.doi.org/10.1016/j.thorsurg.2015.04.006
1547-4127/15/$ – see front matter

are potential candidates for pneumonectomy undergo an appropriate preoperative physiologic assessment to facilitate informed decision-making by both patients and surgeons. The decision regarding a patient's candidacy for a pneumonectomy can then accurately be placed in the context of operative risk. Physiologic assessment should include a thorough preoperative history and physical examination, with specific attention paid to signs and symptoms of cardiopulmonary compromise. Several standardized indices, such as metabolic equivalent tests[6] and the Duke Activity Status Index,[7] have been published. However, a simple review of systems provides an essential, noninvasive means of assessing a patient's functional capacity and risk of perioperative morbidity and mortality. For instance, a patient who reports an inability to walk 4 blocks or to climb 2 flights of stairs without symptomatic limitation has a significantly increased risk of developing perioperative cardiovascular complications following pneumonectomy.[8] Ancillary studies are a critical adjunct, but should not supplant the clinician's general assessment of a patient's physiologic fitness.

Given the relatively high incidence of perioperative arrhythmias and concomitant cardiovascular disease, a preoperative electrocardiogram should be obtained for all patients being considered for pneumonectomy.[9] The thoracic revised cardiac risk index (ThRCRI) is a useful screening tool to identify patients at an increased risk of cardiovascular complications, who may need further preoperative evaluation.[9,10] According the current (2014) American College of Chest Physician Guidelines, patients with a ThRCRI >1.5, with a cardiac condition requiring medications, a newly suspected cardiac condition, or an inability to climb 2 flights of steps should be evaluated by a cardiologist for consideration of further cardiac testing.[9] The authors routinely obtain an echocardiogram on all of their patients being considered for pneumonectomy to assess right and left heart function and to estimate the pulmonary artery pressures (PAPs), to gauge the risk of postpneumonectomy pulmonary hypertension.

In addition to evaluating cardiovascular risk, pulmonary fitness should also be assessed. A baseline assessment of arterial gas exchange is important for future comparison and provides prognostic information. Specifically, preoperative hypoxemia, defined as an arterial oxygen saturation of less than 90% at rest, is associated with an increased risk of postoperative complications.[11] Despite being historically quoted as an exclusion criterion for pulmonary resection, hypercapnia (carbon dioxide partial pressure >45 mm Hg) is not an independent risk factor for perioperative complications. It does, however, indicate a need for further physiologic testing.[12]

Pulmonary function tests also provide essential information regarding the ability of a patient to tolerate a pneumonectomy. A predicted postoperative (PPO) forced expiratory volume in 1 second (FEV_1) greater than 60% and a diffusion capacity of the lung for carbon monoxide (D_{LCO}) >60% indicate a low risk for perioperative complications; further testing is not indicated.[9] For patients with either a PPO FEV_1 or a PPO D_{LCO} less than 60%, an exercise test (eg, stair climb or shuttle walk test) should be performed.[9] Patients with either a PPO FEV_1 or a PPO D_{LCO} less than 30% or who demonstrate poor reserve during an exercise test (eg, walk <25 shuttles on the shuttle walk test or <22 m on the stair climb) are at a high risk for perioperative morbidity and mortality. Such patients should be evaluated with formal cardiopulmonary exercise testing to assess their maximal oxygen consumption (Vo_2 max).[12] Although the threshold has been debated, a Vo_2 max of 15 mL/kg/min or greater indicates sufficient cardiopulmonary reserve. A Vo_2 max less than 10 mL/kg/min is associated with an increased risk of perioperative complications. The care of such patients should be discussed at a multidisciplinary conference and may be best limited to nonoperative treatment options.[13]

Poor cardiopulmonary function may preclude a patient from undergoing pneumonectomy, yet chronologic age alone should not. Lung cancer primarily affects people older than 50, a significant number of whom (30%–35%) are older than 70.[9,14] As the longevity of the general population increases, an increasing number of patients older than 70 will be diagnosed with lung cancer. In fact, the age-adjusted incident rates for lung cancer among patients over the age of 65 increased by 50% from 1975 (about 220 per 100,000 person-years) to 2011 (about 330 per 100,000 person-years).[15] Rather than chronologic age, factors such as tumor stage, comorbidities, performance status, and life expectancy should be taken into consideration when determining whether a patient is a candidate for a pneumonectomy.[9] The increased risk of complications after pneumonectomy in older patients noted in some studies may be confounded by comorbidities. Associated comorbidities may have precluded some older patients from undergoing resection, and others may have refused intervention; nonetheless, a significant proportion may be denied an operation, because of the erroneous assumption that older patients' postoperative life expectancy is too short or that their quality-of-life would be impaired. On the contrary, the life expectancy of a 70-year-old is 14.7 years; of an 80-year-old, 8.8 years.[16] Furthermore, a 75-year-old individual will likely spend about 60% of the rest of his or her life living independently.[17] Thus, a significant number of quality person-years will be lost if physiologically fit older patients are denied an operation. Because the physiologic age and the chronologic age of a patient are often not synchronous, the appropriateness of surgery must be assessed on an individual basis.

An evaluation by a multidisciplinary team, which includes a medical oncologist, radiation oncologist, pulmonologist, cardiologist, and a thoracic surgeon who specializes in lung cancer treatment, can be especially beneficial in higher-risk patients to weigh the survival benefit of a pneumonectomy with curative intent against the risk of perioperative morbidity and mortality.[9] Several studies have demonstrated that patients evaluated by a multidisciplinary team are more likely to receive guideline treatment,[16,18] which ultimately translates into improved survival.

MORTALITY

Early pneumonectomy series were marked by high mortality rates. After the first successful pneumonectomy for lung cancer in 1932,[19] the next 16 pneumonectomies performed by Dr Evarts Graham died in the hospital.[20] Since then, mortalities have steadily declined. Several contemporary series have reported mortalities to be 3% to 5.8% after standard pneumonectomy[3,4,21–24] and 5% to 8.5% after EPP.[22,25–29]

Several studies have identified various independent risk factors for 30-day hospital mortality, including American Society of Anesthesiologists classification,[30,31] congestive heart failure (CHF),[32] coronary artery disease,[31,33,34] prior acute myocardial infarction,[32] diabetes,[34] cerebrovascular disease,[32] chronic renal insufficiency,[32] lower FEV_1,[29,30] malnutrition,[2] high preoperative C-reactive protein levels,[29] intraoperative blood loss (>4 units),[2] intravenous fluid volume,[35] right-sided pneumonectomy,[36] and low-volume centers.[34] Although increasing age has been identified by several studies as a risk factor for 30-day hospital mortality,[2,33,34,36] it is unclear from these studies whether associated comorbidities (which tend to occur at a greater frequency in older patients) are confounding this finding.

After pneumonectomy, patients require careful follow-up; the risk of complications remains significant after discharge from the hospital. In a series of 505 patients undergoing pneumonectomy from 2005 to 2011, more than half of the deaths occurred within the first 90 days after discharge from the hospital,[32] highlighting the importance of careful surveillance after hospital discharge. In the authors' practice, they provide rigorous outpatient care during the first 1 to 4 weeks following discharge from the hospital, including frequent office visits and telephone communications. On some occasions, they will arrange once-weekly or twice-weekly office visits until they are confident in their trajectory.

MORBIDITY

Despite decreasing rates of operative mortality, rates of morbidity after standard pneumonectomy (25%–60%)[2,22–24,33,37,38] and EPP (30%–60%)[29,39] remain significant. Knowledge of risk factors for morbidity after pneumonectomy is important to mitigate the impact of factors that are modifiable and to guide postoperative care. Various studies have identified several independent risk factors for postoperative complications, including age,[2,22] malnutrition (>10% weight loss),[2] cardiovascular disease,[33] CHF,[22] low FEV_1[22,23,37]/chronic obstructive pulmonary disease (COPD),[2] (long) operating room time,[2] acute blood loss anemia,[2,37] and right pneumonectomy.[37]

There has been debate in the literature regarding whether patients who smoke up to the time of surgery do[2,40] or do not[33,41,42] have an increased risk of postoperative complications. Nonetheless, patients should be counseled about the potential risks of continuing to smoke and should be advised to stop smoking irrespective of the timing of pneumonectomy.

There has also been considerable debate whether neoadjuvant therapy does[22,43] or does not[21] increase the risk of complications (including death). One phase III clinical trial of neoadjuvant chemoradiation therapy followed by resection versus definitive chemoradiation therapy for stage IIIa non-small cell lung cancer noted a 27% 30-day mortality for pneumonectomy after neoadjuvant therapy.[44] Nonetheless, a single-institution study that included a high-volume team of dedicated general thoracic surgeons and a systematized approach to patient care demonstrated the pneumonectomy can be performed with an acceptable 30-day mortality (6%) after neoadjuvant chemoradiation therapy.[45]

TECHNICAL COMPLICATIONS

Postoperative Hemorrhage

The incidence of acute blood loss anemia after pneumonectomy is 1% to 4%.[2,29,33] Bleeding can be minimized by meticulous hemostasis, avoiding hypothermia, and correction of any coagulopathy. In addition, the chest should be irrigated at the end of the operation to eliminate the endogenous thrombolytic factors (eg, plasmin) that are innately a component of clotted blood. For patients who undergo EPP, the authors have found argon beam coagulation to be beneficial in reducing chest wall bleeding from the small pleural vessels that are disrupted during an extrapleural dissection. For patients who have ongoing coagulopathy and bleeding despite aggressive corrective measures, consideration should be given to temporarily packing their chest with laparotomy pads for 12 to 24 hours to facilitate resuscitation and correction of coagulopathy in the intensive care unit (ICU).

Patch Complications

Pericardial and diaphragm patch complications occur in 5% of patients undergoing EPP.[29] Pericardial patch complications include an overly constrictive patch that can result in restrictive/tamponade physiology or a poorly secured patch (sewn to the weaker adjacent pericardial tissues rather than the cut edge of the pericardium) that can result in cardiac herniation. Technical errors in diaphragm reconstruction can also result in cardiovascular complications; constriction of the inferior vena cava will impair diastolic filling of the ventricle, and a patch that is constructed too loosely will allow the liver to impinge on the heart and impair venous return when the patient is lying supine.

Dehiscence of the diaphragmatic patch is a technical complication that results in herniation of abdominal viscera into the ipsilateral hemithorax.[46] As a technical point during left EPP, the authors leave a rim of diaphragmatic crus on the esophagus and have noted a decrease in the rate of gastric herniation.[39] The authors' technique of constructing and securing the diaphragmatic patch has also evolved over time. Two polytetrafluoroethylene (PTFE) patches are stapled together to create a dynamic seam in the center that reduces tension on the sutures that secure the patch to the chest wall. With this technique, they have noted a decrease in the rate of patch dehiscence from 12% to 3.8%.[39]

CARDIOVASCULAR COMPLICATIONS

Arrhythmias

Supraventricular arrhythmias are among the most common complications after pneumonectomy, occurring in 4% to 25% of patients following standard pneumonectomy[4,24,33,37,47] and 27% to 44% after EPP.[29,39] The peak incidence is between postoperative day 1 and 4, although it may present as late as 7 to 12 days after surgery.[4]

The mechanisms of postoperative atrial fibrillation are complex and multifactorial and likely involve the presence of an underlying susceptible atrial substrate that is driven into an arrhythmogenic state by aggravating factors (ie, high adrenergic tone after surgery, postoperative systemic inflammatory response, local inflammation of the atrium, and electrolyte abnormalities).[48,49] Risk factors for atrial arrhythmias include age (over the age of 65),[4] right-sided pneumonectomy,[4] intrapericardial dissection,[4] and any major complication.[4]

Based on the 2014 American Association for Thoracic Surgery Guidelines, recommended prevention strategies include continuing β-blockers in patients taking β-blockers before surgery, using intravenous magnesium supplementation if serum magnesium levels are low, using diltiazem in those patients with preserved cardiac function who were not taking β-blockers before surgery, or using amiodarone in patients at an intermediate to high risk of developing postoperative atrial fibrillation.[49]

All patients with new onset atrial fibrillation should be managed by evaluating and treating all possible correctable triggers, by optimizing fluid balance, and by maintaining normal electrolyte levels. Hemodynamically stable patients with new onset atrial fibrillation with a rapid ventricular response should be treated with intravenous β-blockers or non-dihydropyridine calcium channel blockers (ie, diltiazem) to achieve a heart rate of 100 beats per minute or less. Patients that are hemodynamically unstable should undergo direct current cardioversion.[49]

For patients with refractory atrial fibrillation, systemic anticoagulation should be used cautiously; the benefits must be carefully weighed against the risk of bleeding (especially after EPP). The lack of a lung in the hemithorax after standard pneumonectomy or EPP (to tamponade the small parietal vessels that are disrupted during the extrapleural dissection) and the negative pressures generated by the normal mechanics of breathing place these patients at a high risk for a hemothorax. Because 3 to 4 L of blood can occupy a hemithorax, the patient may lose nearly their entire blood volume before the correct diagnosis is made. Consequently, for patients who would otherwise require anticoagulation, consideration should be given to elective cardioversion after excluding the presence of an atrial thrombus via transesophageal echocardiography.

Myocardial Infarction

Coronary artery disease is an independent risk factor for complications after pneumonectomy.[32] The risk of a postoperative myocardial infarction is approximately 0.2% to 2.1% after standard pneumonectomy[2,24,37,47] and 1.5% after EPP.[39] Patients require a careful preoperative assessment to screen for undiagnosed or undertreated coronary artery disease.[9] The American College of Cardiology/American Heart Association guidelines for preoperative coronary revascularization are similar to the general guidelines for revascularization.[50]

For patients who have had prior coronary artery bypass grafting and who later require EPP, care must be taken to avoid injury to an ipsilateral internal mammary artery graft during the extrapleural dissection.

Cardiac Arrest

Cardiac arrest after standard pneumonectomy or EPP is rare (incidence, 3%–7%).[2,39] Several points regarding the management of cardiac arrest after pneumonectomy are noteworthy. Because of the mediastinal shift that occurs after pneumonectomy, the heart cannot be compressed between the sternum and vertebral column during closed chest compressions. As a result, closed chest compressions are futile. Furthermore, if an intrapericardial dissection has been performed, compressions may result in cardiac herniation. Consequently, cardiac arrest within 10 days of pneumonectomy mandates an emergency thoracotomy and open cardiac massage in the ICU. In addition to open massage, emergency thoracotomy allows drainage of any compressive pericardial fluid, release of constrictive pericardial or diaphragmatic patches, or reduction of cardiac herniation (if present). After successful resuscitation, the patient is taken to the operating room for a washout and (if present) correction of any mechanical cause of the arrest.[39] It is imperative that all members of the care team are educated on the appropriate management of this complication to avoid delay in effective resuscitation.

Pulmonary Artery Hypertension

Preoperative pulmonary hypertension is a risk factor for perioperative complications after cardiac and noncardiac surgery.[51,52] Severe pulmonary hypertension (mean PAP, >55 mm Hg) is a contraindication to pneumonectomy. The authors' current preoperative evaluation includes an estimate of a patient's PAP with transthoracic echocardiography taken in the context of his or her relative perfusion to the affected lung noted on a quantitative ventilation/perfusion scan. For instance, a patient with a mean PAP of 25 mm Hg with only 10% perfusion to the affected lung is more likely to be able to tolerate the cardiopulmonary consequences of a pneumonectomy than a patient with a mean PAP of 25 mm Hg and 60% perfusion to the affected lung. The authors use preoperative right heart catheterization selectively, primarily in those patients who are deemed marginal candidates for pneumonectomy based on their PAP estimates from their echocardiogram. In appropriately selected patients for pneumonectomy, the risk of pulmonary hypertension is 30% to 40%. However, most cases of postpneumonectomy pulmonary hypertension (about 80%) are mild and have little impact on functional capacity.[53]

The authors use pulmonary artery catheters selectively in patients who undergo a standard pneumonectomy, primarily when their noninvasive studies suggest that they may not be able to tolerate the increase in right ventricular output to the remaining lung. During the dissection in such patients, the pulmonary artery should be "test" clamped before dividing the hilar structures to assure that the patient will be able to tolerate the hemodynamic effects of a pneumonectomy. Because of the systemic inflammatory response associated with heated intraoperative chemotherapy, the authors place a pulmonary artery catheter in all patients undergoing EPP to guide their perioperative management. For patients who are marginal candidates for EPP, the pulmonary artery should also be test clamped before dividing the hilar structures to assess for changes in PAPs. Patients who have an increase in their mean PAP to 40 mm Hg may be better suited for a pleurectomy than an EPP.

PAP is a function of left atrial pressure (LAP), cardiac output (CO), and pulmonary vascular resistance (PVR):

$$\text{PAP} = \text{LAP} + (\text{CO} \times \text{PVR})/80$$

Consequently, the management of postpneumonectomy pulmonary hypertension is aimed at aggressively treating the underlying cause and optimizing each of these factors. Systemic perfusion must be maintained by optimizing fluid status and by using vasopressors, if needed, to maintain systolic blood pressure. Pulmonary vascular resistance can acutely increase in the setting of hypoxia, hypercapnia, acidosis, increased sympathetic tone (eg, pain), exogenous or endogenous pulmonary vasoconstrictors, or a PE.[54] Pulmonary vasodilators such as dobutamine or prostaglandins may be needed if treating these factors fails to sufficiently reduce right ventricular afterload.[54]

Mechanical Cardiac Complications

Constrictive inflammatory epicarditis

In a series of 328 patients who underwent EPP at the Brigham and Women's Hospital, 2.7%

developed constrictive physiology from inflammatory epicarditis.[39] Interestingly, all cases of constrictive epicarditis occurred after left EPP when the left pericardium was not routinely reconstructed. Most patients required reoperation to remove the scarred epicardial tissue. During the later years of the study (when the left pericardium was routinely reconstructed after EPP), there were no additional cases of epicarditis.

Cardiac herniation

Cardiac herniation, a rare complication after intrapericardial pneumonectomy or EPP, is precipitated by sudden changes in intrathoracic pressure (eg, coughing, placing a pneumonectomy space chest tube to suction, or sudden increases in peak airway pressure during mechanical ventilation).[46] Hemodynamic collapse following a change in patient positioning should heighten the clinical suspicion of cardiac herniation.[55] Following successful resuscitation, the patient is taken back to the operating room (if not already there) for a washout and correction of the cause of herniation.

Because of the risk of cardiac herniation, pericardial reconstruction is mandatory after right intrapericardial pneumonectomy and right EPP. Because the left hemithorax is smaller than the right, pericardial reconstruction is optional after a left intrapericardial pneumonectomy or EPP, although the authors routinely reconstruct the pericardium in such patients. One technical error that increases the risk of herniation is sewing the patch to the weak tissues surrounding the pericardium rather than the pericardium itself. Patients who undergo pleurectomy and partial pericardial resection for mesothelioma do not require pericardial reconstruction because the lung acts as a barrier to cardiac herniation.

Acute mediastinal shift

Rapid fluid evacuation from the pneumonectomy space can cause a mediastinal shift toward the pneumonectomy space, resulting in lung hyperexpansion and impaired cardiac filling. Rapid fluid accumulation into the pneumonectomy space (eg, from hemorrhage, a lymphatic leak or the normal fluid shifts that happen after pneumonectomy), conversely, can cause a mediastinal shift away from the pneumonectomy space, resulting in compression (and impaired ventilation) of the remaining lung. The authors manage the mediastinum with a 14-Fr red rubber catheter, which is connected to a pressure transducer. For men who undergo EPP, the authors remove approximately 1000 cc of air from the pneumonectomy space after a right EPP and 750 cc of air from pneumonectomy space after left EPP while the patient is still in the operating room. For women who undergo EPP, the authors remove approximately 750 cc of air from the pneumonectomy space after a right EPP and 500 cc of air from pneumonectomy space after left EPP while the patient is still in the operating room. While the patient is in the ICU, the authors use the red rubber catheter to keep the mediastinum balanced and to remove fluid if the pneumonectomy space fills too rapidly. If there is an increase in the transmitted pressure, mediastinal shift on radiograph, or a decline in clinical status, fluid is removed.[46,56] This removal of fluid allows a careful balance of the mediastinum dictated by the onset of clinical signs and symptoms and avoids the cardiopulmonary risks of rapidly emptying the pneumonectomy space.

Some surgeons prefer to place a standard chest tube in the pneumonectomy space. If this approach is taken, the suction connector on a traditional atrium should be broken or a balanced drainage system should be used to prevent the risk of mediastinal shift if the chest tube is placed to suction. Alternatively, if there is no bleeding, some surgeons forego chest tube placement and simply aspirate air and fluid out of the pneumonectomy space at the end of the operation.

Tamponade

Tamponade physiology may be the result of either a pericardial effusion or a constrictive patch, resulting in impaired diastolic filling of the ventricle and hemodynamic instability. An important clue in the operative room that an overly constrictive patch is impairing ventricular filling occurs when that patient is turned from the lateral decubitus to the supine position and manifests as persistent hypotension and an increase in filling pressures. The treatment of choice is to re-explore the chest immediately and reconstruct the pericardium with a looser patch.[39]

RESPIRATORY COMPLICATIONS

Respiratory complications (eg, aspiration, pneumonia, and acute respiratory distress syndrome [ARDS]) are a frequent source of morbidity and mortality after standard pneumonectomy or EPP (range, 16%–40%).[33,39,47,57] Because pulmonary reserve is limited after pneumonectomy, respiratory complications are life-threatening. As such, they should be proactively prevented and aggressively treated. Many of these complications are closely related to vocal cord paralysis. In fact, recurrent laryngeal nerve injury complicates 1.5% to 5.3%[24,37] of standard pneumonectomies and 6.3% of EPPs.[39] Because vocal dysfunction results in poor pulmonary toilet and a high risk of aspiration, the authors have adopted a practice of early vocal fold medialization by their otolaryngology colleagues and have noted improved outcomes with this approach.[58]

Pneumonia

Pneumonia after pneumonectomy is a life-threatening complication that has been reported in 2% to 10% of patients in large series.[24,29,33,37,47] Pneumonia is often the result of poor pulmonary toilet, which is exacerbated by poor pain control and immobility or prolonged mechanical ventilation. Volume overload is often a contributing factor. To lessen the risk of pneumonia, the authors' practice includes preoperative smoking cessation, early (and frequent) ambulation postoperatively, chest physiotherapy by nurses and respiratory therapists, aggressive diuresis, treatment of postthoracotomy pain, and frequent toilet bronchoscopy for retained secretions.

Patients who develop pneumonia despite these efforts should be treated with appropriate antibiotics based on bronchoalveolar culture data and ongoing treatment of factors that may have precipitated pneumonia (eg, poor pulmonary toilet, immobility, poor pain control, volume overload, and aspiration).

Acute Respiratory Distress Syndrome

ARDS is characterized by onset of worsening respiratory symptoms within a week of a clinical insult, diffuse opacities not explained by effusions or atelectasis, and noncardiogenic pulmonary edema. ARDS is classified (according to the Berlin definition) as mild ($200< Pao_2/Fio_2 \leq 300$ on positive end-expiratory pressure [PEEP] $\geq$5 cm H_2O), moderate ($100< Pao_2/Fio_2 \leq 200$ on PEEP $\geq$5 cm H_2O), and severe ($Pao_2/Fio_2 \leq 100$ on PEEP $\geq$5 cm H_2O).[59] The term "acute lung injury" (Pao_2/Fio_2 $\leq$300) is no longer recognized by the Berlin definition, although it still appears in the thoracic surgery literature. The term "post-pneumonectomy pulmonary edema" is also synonymous with ARDS.[2,33,60,61] ARDS occurs in 2.7% to 3.1% of patients after standard pneumonectomy[24,38,62] and in 1% to 3.6% patients after EPP.[29,39] Not surprisingly, mortality from ARDS after pneumonectomy is 50% to 70%.[62–64]

Capillary endothelial injury and increased permeability resulting in the accumulation of protein-rich fluid in the interstitium is a cardinal feature of ARDS.[65] Potential causative factors include volutrauma[66] and hyperoxia[67] during intraoperative single-lung ventilation, blood product transfusion,[68] occult infection, occult aspiration, and unrecognized microemboli. Sheer stress from volume overload may be important[66]; this may explain why some studies have identified poor postoperative predicted lung function as a risk factor for postoperative ARDS.[60,69] Consequently, patients with relatively low perfusion to the remaining lung (noted on a preoperative quantitative ventilation/perfusion scan) may not be able to accommodate the increase in CO to that lung after pneumonectomy because of the associated increase in pulmonary vascular pressure and sheer forces on the endothelium.

As compared with endothelial injury, the contribution of alveolar injury to the pathophysiology of ARDS is poorly understood but likely plays an important role as well.[65] Potential mechanisms of alveolar injury include infection, aspiration, volutrauma, and unbalanced chest drainage.[70]

Treatment of ARDS is supportive. Potential uncorrected causative factors (eg, infection) should be sought out and addressed. Mechanical ventilation with lung-protective strategies (tidal volumes, 6 mg/kg ideal body weight) should be used to minimize volutrauma.[71] The Fio_2 should be decreased to the lowest tolerated level to minimize oxidative trauma. Fluid should be restricted, and the patient should be aggressively diuresed. Although there is no convincing benefit based on the available evidence, inhaled nitric oxide is often used.[72] For patients with severe ARDS, early prone positioning should be considered.[73] There is no evidence that corticosteroids improve outcomes in patients with ARDS and may actually be associated with worse outcomes.[74]

Prevention of ARDS is a more effective strategy than treatment. Proactive measures in the operating room include minimizing volutrauma during single-lung isolation and using the lowest Fio_2 tolerated. Perioperative fluid administration should be minimized, and the patient should be aggressively diuresed (with vasopressor support if needed). Pulmonary toilet should be aggressive. The risk of aspiration should be assessed for each patient and any contributing factors to aspiration (eg, mental status changes, vocal cord dysfunction, and deconditioning) should be addressed.

Postpneumonectomy Syndrome

Postpneumonectomy syndrome is a rare, late complication that occurs years following right pneumonectomy. The syndrome is caused by severe shift of the mediastinum to the right (**Fig. 1**), resulting in tracheal deviation posteriorly, to the right, and then back anteriorly and to the left. As

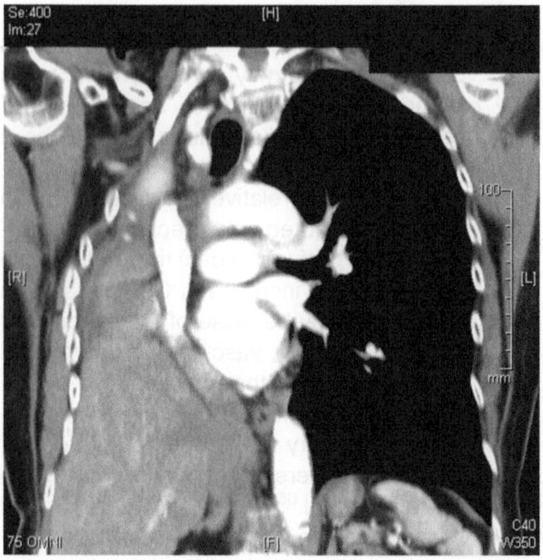

Fig. 1. Severe mediastinal shift in the setting of postpneumonectomy syndrome after a right pneumonectomy. (*Courtesy of* Shanda H. Blackmon, MD, MPH, Rochester, MN.)

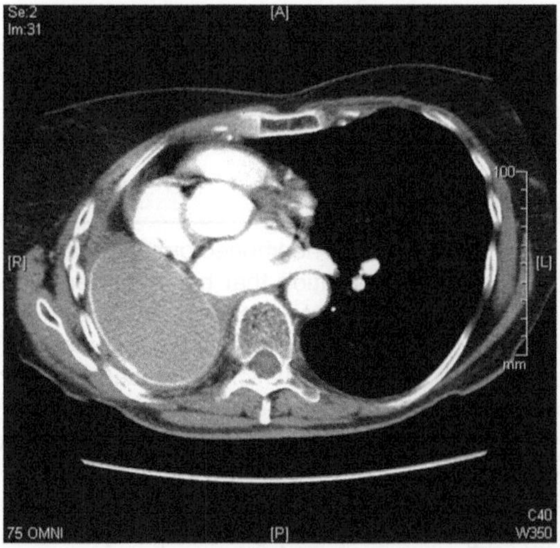

Fig. 2. Use of an expandable prosthesis for postpneumonectomy syndrome. (*Courtesy of* Shanda H. Blackmon, MD, MPH, Rochester, MN.)

a result, the left main-stem bronchus is compressed between the spinal column and the left pulmonary artery, and the left lower lobe bronchus is kinked between the aorta and pulmonary artery. As a result of the distorted anatomy of the trachea and left-sided airways, ventilation is impaired. Stretching of the airways results in secondary tracheobronchomalacia due to destruction of the myoelastic elements that provide support for the cartilaginous portion of the airways.[75] The syndrome presents as decreased exercise capacity, increased work of breathing, and inspiratory stridor.[75] Several techniques have been used to fill the right pneumonectomy space to either prevent or treat the mediastinal shift, including filling the right pleural space with Lucite balls, dividing the phrenic nerve, and implantation of an expandable prosthesis (**Fig. 2**).[75]

EMPYEMA

Empyema has been reported following 1.3% to 5.6% of standard pneumonectomies[33,37,38] and 2.4% to 14% of EPPs.[29,39] The management of a postpneumonectomy empyema depends on the timing of presentation. Patients who present in the first month after pneumonectomy can often be managed by a thoracoscopic debridement of the pleural space and washout followed by postoperative irrigation with antibiotics for 5 days.[39,76] For patients who present with an empyema in the first few weeks after EPP with a degree of infection too advanced for thoracoscopic washout, the authors' practice is for an early Clagett window, with removal of the PTFE pericardial and diaphragmatic patches in a staged fashion due to the risk of herniation of the heart or abdominal contents if these patches are removed too early. After 2 to 4 weeks of dressing changes, the mediastinum is usually sufficiently scarred in to allow removal of the pericardial patch without the risk of cardiac herniation. At this same time, a right-sided diaphragmatic patch can also be removed because the liver and postoperative scarring at 4 weeks provides an effective barrier against herniation of abdominal viscera. For left-sided diaphragmatic patches, consideration may be given to replacing the PTFE patch with a biological mesh 4 weeks after EPP if there is concern for a high risk of abdominal viscera herniation.

For patients who present months to years after pneumonectomy or EPP with an empyema, open thoracostomy is often required with either a Clagett window or an Eloesser flap (**Fig. 3**), followed by pedicled muscle flap coverage once the infection clears.

Bronchopleural Fistula

Bronchopleural fistula (BPF) is a rare but life-threatening complication after pneumonectomy (incidence, 1.7%–11%)[24,30,33,37,38,77] and EPP (incidence, 0.6%–8%).[29,39] The mortality associated with a BPF is high (up to 40%). Risk factors for BPF include immunosuppression (including steroids and preoperative chemotherapy), diabetes, anemia, COPD, malnutrition, a long (>2 cm) bronchial stump, preoperative radiation

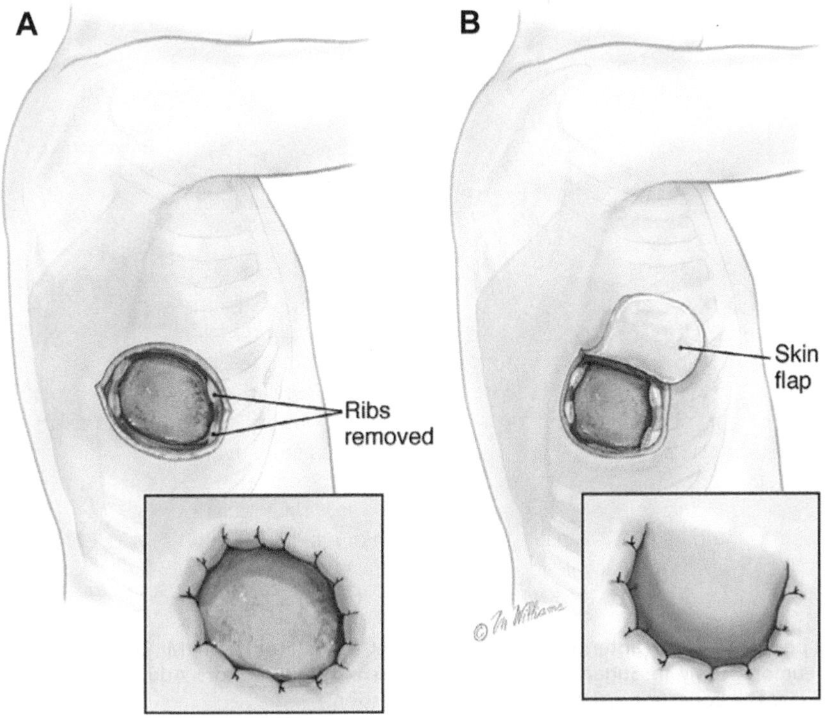

Fig. 3. Clagett window (*A*) and Eloesser flap (*B*). (*From* Jaklitsch MT. Thoracic incisions. In: Sugarbaker D, Bueno R, Colson Y, et al, editors. Adult chest surgery. 2nd edition. New York: McGraw-Hill Education; 2015. p. 17; with permission.)

therapy, right pneumonectomy, completion pneumonectomy, and devascularization of the bronchial stump.[78] Minimizing modifiable risk factors (eg, ensuring adequate nutrition, avoid leaving a long bronchial stump, and avoid devascularizing the bronchial blood supply during the dissection) will minimize the risk of BPF.

Several investigators have explored endobronchial management of BPFs including ethanol injection into the submucosa of the fistula,[79] fibrin glue,[80] and albumin-glutaraldehyde tissue adhesive (BioGlue; Cryolife, Kennesaw, GA).[81] There is no evidence to support the superiority of one compound over the other.[82] These compounds are likely best suited for small (<1 mm) BPFs or for BPFs that are less than 5 mm as a temporizing maneuver before definitive treatment. The use of stents to exclude a BPF is in its infancy.[83,84]

The authors prefer to manage a BPF in 2 stages, beginning with source control and nutritional support followed by fistula control and pleural space obliteration. Upon admission, the authors place a chest tube for temporary source control. In general, patients with a BPF require an open thoracostomy to prevent contamination of the remaining lung and aggressive toilet bronchoscopy of any aspirated secretions to minimize the risk of pneumonia. Wet-to-dry thoracostomy dressing changes are performed every 8 to 12 hours, and the patient is placed on broad-spectrum antibiotics. Adequate nutrition is essential to maximize the chance of successfully managing the acute infection and closing the BPF once the infection has cleared. Many of these patients require a jejunostomy tube to facilitate meeting their nutritional needs. In general, for patients who require enteric nutritional support after pneumonectomy or EPP, the authors prefer to feed the jejunum (rather than the stomach) due to the risk of aspiration with gastric feeds. Once the pleural space is clean, the fistula is closed with a pedicled muscle flap (**Fig. 4**)[85] or omentum (**Fig. 5**).[86] The authors prefer to obliterate the pleural space with a muscle transposition. Others have had success obliterating the pleural space with thoracoplasty[87] or filling the space with antibiotic containing solution (ie, Clagett procedure).[88]

HEMATOLOGIC COMPLICATIONS

Deep venous thrombosis (DVT; incidence, 1.5%–6.4%[2,37,39]) and pulmonary embolus (PE; incidence, 0.5%–4%[2,24,33,37,39]) are important

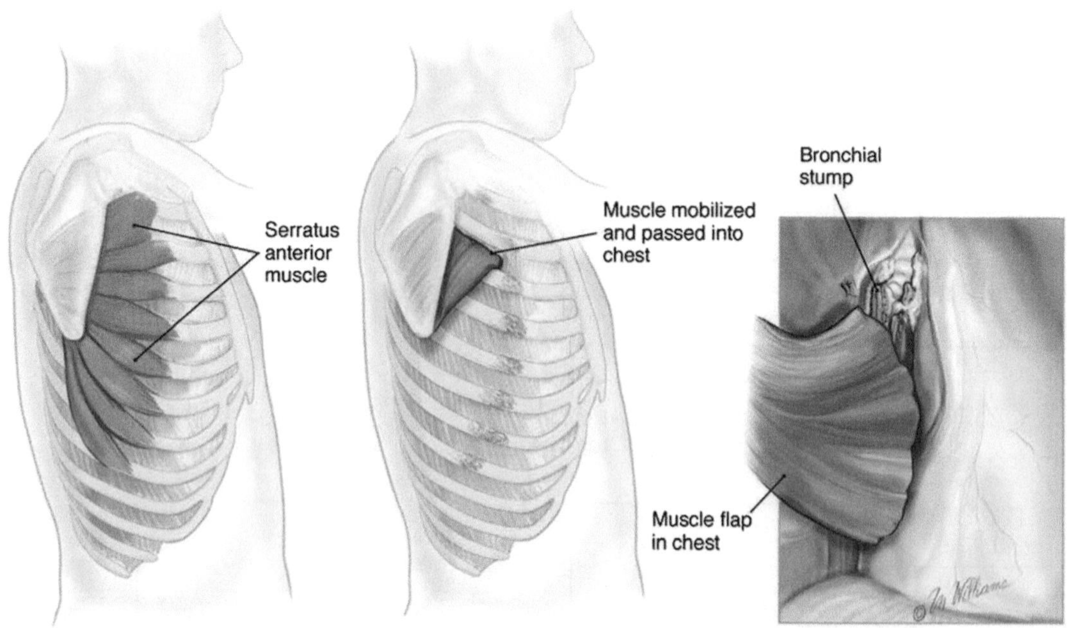

Fig. 4. Use of a pedicled serratus anterior muscle flap to cover a BPF. (*From* Berry MF, Harpole DH. Bronchopleural fistula after pneumonectomy. In: Sugarbaker D, Bueno R, Colson Y, et al, editors. Adult chest surgery. 2nd edition. New York: McGraw-Hill Education; 2015. p. 683; with permission.)

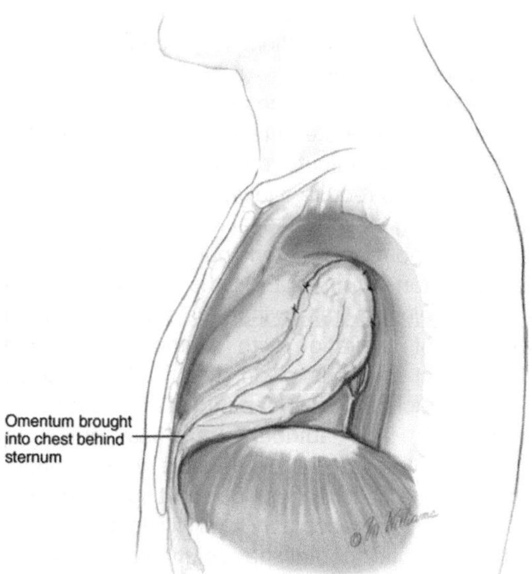

Fig. 5. Use of an omental flap to cover a BPF. (*From* Berry MF, Harpole DH. Bronchopleural fistula after pneumonectomy. In: Sugarbaker D, Bueno R, Colson Y, et al, editors. Adult chest surgery. 2nd edition. New York: McGraw-Hill Education; 2015. p. 683; with permission.)

complications to recognize early after pneumonectomy. In particular, PE is associated with a high mortality rate in patients after pneumonectomy. In a series of 328 EPPs at the Brigham and Women's Hospital, PE was the most common cause of 30-day mortality, accounting for 30% of all deaths.[39] In another multi-institutional series of 251 EPPs, PE was also noted as the most frequent cause of death in their cohort.[29]

Because a PE to the remaining lung is always life-threatening after pneumonectomy, the authors have adopted an aggressive proactive approach to prevention and treatment. In addition to routine subcutaneous prophylaxis (with either unfractionated heparin or low-molecular-weight heparin) and pneumatic compression devices, the authors routinely screen all patients preoperatively and at 5- to 7-day intervals during their hospital stay for DVTs using lower-extremity duplex ultrasound. If a DVT is identified preoperatively, an inferior vena cava filter is placed. If one is identified postoperatively, the authors treat above-the-knee DVTs with systemic anticoagulation. However, systemic anticoagulation following pneumonectomy (especially after EPP) should be used with caution in the early postoperative period because of a risk of spontaneous bleeding. In the absence of the lung to tamponade bleeding from the chest wall, catastrophic blood loss can occur into the pneumonectomy space before the correct diagnosis is made.

SUMMARY

Although mortality rates after pneumonectomy have steadily declined over the last 80 years, morbidity rates remain significant. Patients with pneumonectomy live along a narrow margin of error given their limited cardiopulmonary reserve. Consequently, proactive approaches to patient selection and to mitigating potential factors in the perioperative period that contribute to complications are essential components of optimizing outcomes. When complications do occur, they must be aggressively treated to curtail their potential impact on the patient.

REFERENCES

1. Ginsberg RJ, Hill LD, Eagan RT, et al. Modern thirty-day operative mortality for surgical resections in lung cancer. J Thorac Cardiovasc Surg 1983;86(5): 654–8.
2. Harpole DH Jr, DeCamp MM Jr, Daley J, et al. Prognostic models of thirty-day mortality and morbidity after major pulmonary resection. J Thorac Cardiovasc Surg 1999;117(5):969–79.
3. Allen MS, Darling GE, Pechet TT, et al. Morbidity and mortality of major pulmonary resections in patients with early-stage lung cancer: initial results of the randomized, prospective ACOSOG Z0030 trial. Ann Thorac Surg 2006;81(3):1013–9 [discussion: 1019–20].
4. Harpole DH, Liptay MJ, DeCamp MM Jr, et al. Prospective analysis of pneumonectomy: risk factors for major morbidity and cardiac dysrhythmias. Ann Thorac Surg 1996;61(3):977–82.
5. Rueth NM, Parsons HM, Habermann EB, et al. The long-term impact of surgical complications after resection of stage I nonsmall cell lung cancer: a population-based survival analysis. Ann Surg 2011; 254(2):368–74.
6. Eagle KA, Berger PB, Calkins H, et al. ACC/AHA guideline update for perioperative cardiovascular evaluation for noncardiac surgery—executive summary a report of the American College of Cardiology/American Heart Association Task Force on Practice Guidelines (Committee to Update the 1996 Guidelines on Perioperative Cardiovascular Evaluation for Noncardiac Surgery). Circulation 2002;105(10):1257–67.
7. Hlatky MA, Boineau RE, Higginbotham MB, et al. A brief self-administered questionnaire to determine functional capacity (the Duke Activity Status Index). Am J Cardiol 1989;64(10):651–4.
8. Reilly DF, McNeely MJ, Doerner D, et al. Self-reported exercise tolerance and the risk of serious perioperative complications. Arch Intern Med 1999; 159(18):2185–92.
9. Brunelli A, Kim AW, Berger KI, et al. Physiologic evaluation of the patient with lung cancer being considered for resectional surgery: diagnosis and management of lung cancer, 3rd ed: American College of Chest Physicians evidence-based clinical practice guidelines. Chest 2013;143(5 Suppl): e166S–190S.
10. Brunelli A, Varela G, Salati M, et al. Recalibration of the revised cardiac risk index in lung resection candidates. Ann Thorac Surg 2010;90(1):199–203.
11. Ninan M, Sommers KE, Landreneau RJ, et al. Standardized exercise oximetry predicts postpneumonectomy outcome. Ann Thorac Surg 1997;64(2): 328–32 [discussion: 332–3].
12. Beckles MA, Spiro SG, Colice GL, et al. The physiologic evaluation of patients with lung cancer being considered for resectional surgery. Chest 2003; 123(1 Suppl):105S–14S.
13. British Thoracic Society, Society of Cardiothoracic Surgeons of Great Britain and Ireland Working Party. BTS guidelines: guidelines on the selection of patients with lung cancer for surgery. Thorax 2001; 56(2):89–108.
14. Jemal A, Siegel R, Ward E, et al. Cancer statistics, 2006. CA Cancer J Clin 2006;56(2):106–30.
15. Surveillance epidemiology, and end results (SEER) Program (www.seer.cancer.gov) SEER*stat database: incidence - SEEr 9 regs public-use, Nov 2013 Sub (1973-2011 varying), National Cancer Institute, DCCPS, surveillance research program, cancer statistics branch, released April 2014, based on the November 2013 submission.
16. Freeman RK, Van Woerkom JM, Vyverberg A, et al. The effect of a multidisciplinary thoracic malignancy conference on the treatment of patients with lung cancer. Eur J Cardiothorac Surg 2010;38(1):1–5.
17. Katz S, Branch LG, Branson MH, et al. Active life expectancy. N Engl J Med 1983;309(20):1218–24.
18. Boxer MM, Vinod SK, Shafiq J, et al. Do multidisciplinary team meetings make a difference in the management of lung cancer? Cancer 2011;117(22): 5112–20.
19. Graham EA, Singer JJ. Successful removal of the entire lung for carcinoma of the bronchus. JAMA 1933;101(18):1371–4.
20. Mueller CB. Evarts A. Graham: the life, lives, and times of the surgical spirit of St. Louis. Hamilton (Canada): BC Decker Inc; 2002.
21. Perrot E, Guibert B, Mulsant P, et al. Preoperative chemotherapy does not increase complications after nonsmall cell lung cancer resection. Ann Thorac Surg 2005;80(2):423–7.
22. Shapiro M, Swanson SJ, Wright CD, et al. Predictors of major morbidity and mortality after pneumonectomy utilizing the society for thoracic surgeons general thoracic surgery database. Ann Thorac Surg 2010;90(3):927–34 [discussion: 934–5].

23. Mitsudomi T, Mizoue T, Yoshimatsu T, et al. Postoperative complications after pneumonectomy for treatment of lung cancer: multivariate analysis. J Surg Oncol 1996;61(3):218–22.
24. Darling GE, Abdurahman A, Yi QL, et al. Risk of a right pneumonectomy: role of bronchopleural fistula. Ann Thorac Surg 2005;79(2):433–7.
25. Sugarbaker DJ, Richards WG, Bueno R. Extrapleural pneumonectomy in the treatment of epithelioid malignant pleural mesothelioma: novel prognostic implications of combined N1 and N2 nodal involvement based on experience in 529 patients. Ann Surg 2014;260(4):577–80 [discussion: 580–2].
26. Schipper PH, Nichols FC, Thomse KM, et al. Malignant pleural mesothelioma: surgical management in 285 patients. Ann Thorac Surg 2008;85(1):257–64 [discussion: 264].
27. Rice DC, Stevens CW, Correa AM, et al. Outcomes after extrapleural pneumonectomy and intensity-modulated radiation therapy for malignant pleural mesothelioma. Ann Thorac Surg 2007;84(5):1685–92 [discussion: 1692–3].
28. Rusch VW, Rosenzweig K, Venkatraman E, et al. A phase II trial of surgical resection and adjuvant high-dose hemithoracic radiation for malignant pleural mesothelioma. J Thorac Cardiovasc Surg 2001;122(4):788–95.
29. Lauk O, Hoda MA, de Perrot M, et al. Extrapleural pneumonectomy after induction chemotherapy: perioperative outcome in 251 mesothelioma patients from three high-volume institutions. Ann Thorac Surg 2014;98(5):1748–54.
30. Groenendijk RP, Croiset van Uchelen FA, Mol SJ, et al. Factors related to outcome after pneumonectomy: retrospective study of 62 patients. Eur J Surg 1999;165(3):193–7.
31. Licker M, de Perrot M, Hohn L, et al. Perioperative mortality and major cardio-pulmonary complications after lung surgery for non-small cell carcinoma. Eur J Cardiothorac Surg 1999;15(3):314–9.
32. Schneider L, Farrokhyar F, Schieman C, et al. Pneumonectomy: the burden of death after discharge and predictors of surgical mortality. Ann Thorac Surg 2014;98(6):1976–81.
33. Bernard A, Deschamps C, Allen MS, et al. Pneumonectomy for malignant disease: factors affecting early morbidity and mortality. J Thorac Cardiovasc Surg 2001;121(6):1076–82.
34. Romano PS, Mark DH. Patient and hospital characteristics related to in-hospital mortality after lung cancer resection. Chest 1992;101(5):1332–7.
35. Swartz DE, Lachapelle K, Sampalis J, et al. Perioperative mortality after pneumonectomy: analysis of risk factors and review of the literature. Can J Surg 1997;40(6):437–44.
36. van Meerbeeck JP, Damhuis RA, Vos de Wael ML. High postoperative risk after pneumonectomy in elderly patients with right-sided lung cancer. Eur Respir J 2002;19(1):141–5.
37. Martin J, Ginsberg RJ, Abolhoda A, et al. Morbidity and mortality after neoadjuvant therapy for lung cancer: the risks of right pneumonectomy. Ann Thorac Surg 2001;72(4):1149–54.
38. Mansour Z, Kochetkova EA, Santelmo N, et al. Risk factors for early mortality and morbidity after pneumonectomy: a reappraisal. Ann Thorac Surg 2009; 88(6):1737–43.
39. Sugarbaker DJ, Jaklitsch MT, Bueno R, et al. Prevention, early detection, and management of complications after 328 consecutive extrapleural pneumonectomies. J Thorac Cardiovasc Surg 2004;128(1):138–46.
40. Mason DP, Subramanian S, Nowicki ER, et al. Impact of smoking cessation before resection of lung cancer: a Society of Thoracic Surgeons General Thoracic Surgery Database Study. Ann Thorac Surg 2009;88(2):362–70 [discussion: 370–1].
41. Groth SS, Whitson BA, Kuskowski MA, et al. Impact of preoperative smoking status on postoperative complication rates and pulmonary function test results 1-year following pulmonary resection for non-small cell lung cancer. Lung Cancer 2009;64(3): 352–7.
42. Barrera R, Shi W, Amar D, et al. Smoking and timing of cessation: impact on pulmonary complications after thoracotomy. Chest 2005;127(6):1977–83.
43. Doddoli C, Barlesi F, Trousse D, et al. One hundred consecutive pneumonectomies after induction therapy for non-small cell lung cancer: an uncertain balance between risks and benefits. J Thorac Cardiovasc Surg 2005;130(2):416–25.
44. Albain KS, Swann RS, Rusch VW, et al. Radiotherapy plus chemotherapy with or without surgical resection for stage III non-small-cell lung cancer: a phase III randomised controlled trial. Lancet 2009; 374(9687):379–86.
45. Allen AM, Mentzer SJ, Yeap BY, et al. Pneumonectomy after chemoradiation: the Dana-Farber Cancer Institute/Brigham and Women's Hospital experience. Cancer 2008;112(5):1106–13.
46. Zellos L, Jaklitsch MT, Al-Mourgi MA, et al. Complications of extrapleural pneumonectomy. Semin Thorac Cardiovasc Surg 2007;19(4):355–9.
47. Licker M, Spiliopoulos A, Frey JG, et al. Risk factors for early mortality and major complications following pneumonectomy for non-small cell carcinoma of the lung. Chest 2002;121(6):1890–7.
48. Amar D. Perioperative atrial tachyarrhythmias. Anesthesiology 2002;97(6):1618–23.
49. Frendl G, Sodickson AC, Chung MK, et al. 2014 AATS guidelines for the prevention and management of perioperative atrial fibrillation and flutter for thoracic surgical procedures. Executive summary. J Thorac Cardiovasc Surg 2014;148(3):772–91.

50. Fleisher LA, Fleischmann KE, Auerbach AD, et al. 2014 ACC/AHA guideline on perioperative cardiovascular evaluation and management of patients undergoing noncardiac surgery: a report of the American College of Cardiology/American Heart Association task force on practice guidelines. Circulation 2014;130(24):2215–45.
51. Ramakrishna G, Sprung J, Ravi BS, et al. Impact of pulmonary hypertension on the outcomes of noncardiac surgery: predictors of perioperative morbidity and mortality. J Am Coll Cardiol 2005; 45(10):1691–9.
52. Lai HC, Wang KY, Lee WL, et al. Severe pulmonary hypertension complicates postoperative outcome of non-cardiac surgery. Br J Anaesth 2007;99(2): 184–90.
53. Deslauriers J, Ugalde P, Miro S, et al. Adjustments in cardiorespiratory function after pneumonectomy: results of the pneumonectomy project. J Thorac Cardiovasc Surg 2011;141(1):7–15.
54. Minai OA, Yared JP, Kaw R, et al. Perioperative risk and management in patients with pulmonary hypertension. Chest 2013;144(1):329–40.
55. Chambers N, Walton S, Pearce A. Cardiac herniation following pneumonectomy–an old complication revisited. Anaesth Intensive Care 2005;33(3):403–9.
56. Wolf AS, Jacobson FL, Tilleman TR, et al. Managing the pneumonectomy space after extrapleural pneumonectomy: postoperative intrathoracic pressure monitoring. Eur J Cardiothorac Surg 2010;37(4): 770–5.
57. Rostad H, Strand TE, Naalsund A, et al. Lung cancer surgery: the first 60 days. A population-based study. Eur J Cardiothorac Surg 2006;29(5):824–8.
58. Bhattacharyya N, Batirel H, Swanson SJ. Improved outcomes with early vocal fold medialization for vocal fold paralysis after thoracic surgery. Auris Nasus Larynx 2003;30(1):71–5.
59. Ranieri VM, Rubenfeld GD, Thompson BT, et al. Acute respiratory distress syndrome: the Berlin definition. JAMA 2012;307(23):2526–33.
60. Parquin F, Marchal M, Mehiri S, et al. Post-pneumonectomy pulmonary edema: analysis and risk factors. Eur J Cardiothorac Surg 1996;10(11):929–32 [discussion: 933].
61. Jordan S, Mitchell JA, Quinlan GJ, et al. The pathogenesis of lung injury following pulmonary resection. Eur Respir J 2000;15(4):790–9.
62. Kutlu CA, Williams EA, Evans TW, et al. Acute lung injury and acute respiratory distress syndrome after pulmonary resection. Ann Thorac Surg 2000;69(2): 376–80.
63. Tang SS, Redmond K, Griffiths M, et al. The mortality from acute respiratory distress syndrome after pulmonary resection is reducing: a 10-year single institutional experience. Eur J Cardiothorac Surg 2008; 34(4):898–902.
64. Dulu A, Pastores SM, Park B, et al. Prevalence and mortality of acute lung injury and ARDS after lung resection. Chest 2006;130(1):73–8.
65. Matthay MA, Ware LB, Zimmerman GA. The acute respiratory distress syndrome. J Clin Invest 2012; 122(8):2731–40.
66. Licker M, de Perrot M, Spiliopoulos A, et al. Risk factors for acute lung injury after thoracic surgery for lung cancer. Anesth Analg 2003;97(6):1558–65.
67. Fracica PJ, Knapp MJ, Piantadosi CA, et al. Responses of baboons to prolonged hyperoxia: physiology and qualitative pathology. J Appl Physiol (1985) 1991;71(6):2352–62.
68. Vlaar AP, Juffermans NP. Transfusion-related acute lung injury: a clinical review. Lancet 2013; 382(9896):984–94.
69. Alam N, Park BJ, Wilton A, et al. Incidence and risk factors for lung injury after lung cancer resection. Ann Thorac Surg 2007;84(4):1085–91 [discussion: 1091].
70. Alvarez JM, Panda RK, Newman MA, et al. Postpneumonectomy pulmonary edema. J Cardiothorac Vasc Anesth 2003;17(3):388–95.
71. Ventilation with lower tidal volumes as compared with traditional tidal volumes for acute lung injury and the acute respiratory distress syndrome. The Acute Respiratory Distress Syndrome Network. N Engl J Med 2000;342(18):1301–8.
72. Afshari A, Brok J, Moller AM, et al. Inhaled nitric oxide for acute respiratory distress syndrome (ARDS) and acute lung injury in children and adults. Cochrane Database Syst Rev 2010;(7):CD002787.
73. Guerin C, Reignier J, Richard JC, et al. Prone positioning in severe acute respiratory distress syndrome. N Engl J Med 2013;368(23):2159–68.
74. Steinberg KP, Hudson LD, Goodman RB, et al. Efficacy and safety of corticosteroids for persistent acute respiratory distress syndrome. N Engl J Med 2006;354(16):1671–84.
75. Jansen JP, Brutel de la Riviere A, Alting MP, et al. Postpneumonectomy syndrome in adulthood. Surgical correction using an expandable prosthesis. Chest 1992;101(4):1167–70.
76. Hollaus PH, Lax F, Wurnig PN, et al. Videothoracoscopic debridement of the postpneumonectomy space in empyema. Eur J Cardiothorac Surg 1999; 16(3):283–6.
77. Jichen QV, Chen G, Jiang G, et al. Risk factor comparison and clinical analysis of early and late bronchopleural fistula after non-small cell lung cancer surgery. Ann Thorac Surg 2009;88(5):1589–93.
78. Ng CS, Wan S, Lee TW, et al. Post-pneumonectomy empyema: current management strategies. ANZ J Surg 2005;75(7):597–602.
79. Takaoka K, Inoue S, Ohira S. Central bronchopleural fistulas closed by bronchoscopic injection of absolute ethanol. Chest 2002;122(1):374–8.

80. Glover W, Chavis TV, Daniel TM, et al. Fibrin glue application through the flexible fiberoptic bronchoscope: closure of bronchopleural fistulas. J Thorac Cardiovasc Surg 1987;93(3):470–2.
81. Lin J, Iannettoni MD. Closure of bronchopleural fistulas using albumin-glutaraldehyde tissue adhesive. Ann Thorac Surg 2004;77(1):326–8.
82. Lois M, Noppen M. Bronchopleural fistulas: an overview of the problem with special focus on endoscopic management. Chest 2005;128(6):3955–65.
83. Kutlu CA, Patlakoglu S, Tasci AE, et al. A novel technique for bronchopleural fistula closure: an hourglass-shaped stent. J Thorac Cardiovasc Surg 2009;137(1):e46–7.
84. Dutau H, Breen DP, Gomez C, et al. The integrated place of tracheobronchial stents in the multidisciplinary management of large post-pneumonectomy fistulas: our experience using a novel customised conical self-expandable metallic stent. Eur J Cardiothorac Surg 2011;39(2):185–9.
85. Pairolero PC, Arnold PG, Trastek VF, et al. Postpneumonectomy empyema. The role of intrathoracic muscle transposition. J Thorac Cardiovasc Surg 1990;99(6):958–66 [discussion: 966–8].
86. Schneiter D, Cassina P, Korom S, et al. Accelerated treatment for early and late postpneumonectomy empyema. Ann Thorac Surg 2001;72(5):1668–72.
87. Stefani A, Jouni R, Alifano M, et al. Thoracoplasty in the current practice of thoracic surgery: a single-institution 10-year experience. Ann Thorac Surg 2011;91(1):263–8.
88. Zaheer S, Allen MS, Cassivi SD, et al. Postpneumonectomy empyema: results after the Clagett procedure. Ann Thorac Surg 2006;82(1):279–86 [discussion: 286–7].

Video-Assisted Thoracic Surgery After Median Sternotomy for Cardiac Surgery

Derek Serna-Gallegos, MD, Heather Merry, MD,
Robert J. McKenna Jr, MD*

KEYWORDS

• Intraoperative crisis • Mammary artery graft • VATS lobectomy complications

KEY POINTS

- Video-assisted thoracic surgery (VATS) lobectomies can be safely performed in patients with ipsilateral internal mammary artery (IMA) grafts in institutions with cardiopulmonary bypass available to perform redo coronary artery bypass or revision of bypass grafts if an injury to a coronary artery graft does occur.
- Preoperative work-up should include cardiac clearance.
- Cardiac surgery through a median sternotomy usually causes adhesions between the upper lobe and the mediastinum; such adhesions should be lysed carefully to avoid damage to the heart and IMA graft. If the proper plane is not clear, to avoid the IMA graft, the upper lobe parenchyma should be transected to leave some of the lung tissue attached to the mediastinum.
- Injuries to IMA grafts can potentially be managed with primary repair.

INTRODUCTION: NATURE OF THE PROBLEM

The use of video-assisted thoracic surgery (VATS) has steadily increased since its inception in 1992. VATS lobectomy is now a standard approach for early stage 1 lung cancer.[1,2] According to Society of Thoracic Surgeons database information, the rate of VATS lobectomy increased from 21.6% in 2004 to 32% in 2006 to 44.7% in 2010.[3] Regarding the use of VATS for lobectomy, some thoracic surgeons still have concerns about management of intrathoracic adhesions and especially pleural symphysis. Adhesions may lead to difficulty recognizing anatomy or mobilizing the lung from the mediastinum, and thus adhesions may be an indication to convert to a thoracotomy. However, adhesions are not an absolute contraindication to a VATS approach.

The upper lobes are usually adhesed to the mediastinum after median sternotomy for cardiac surgery, especially when the internal mammary artery (IMA) has been harvested for use as a bypass graft. It has long been recognized that the left IMA (LIMA) is at risk of injury during repeat sternotomy, because it can become adherent to the sternum and is displaced to the midline.[4] In the cardiac surgery literature, preoperative computed tomography (CT) scan to identify areas in the mediastinum that appear to be adherent to surrounding structures has been shown to decrease the incidence of re-entry graft injury and subsequently in-hospital mortality.[5]

In addition to looking at the lung mass and the nodes, a thoracic surgeon may review the patient's chest CT scan to look at the relationship of the upper lobes to the IMA graft and mediastinum. CT with contrast can assess the patency of an IMA graft and provide a roadmap for the location of the graft within the anterior

The authors have nothing to disclose.
Division of Thoracic Surgery, Department of Surgery, Cedars-Sinai Medical Center, 8631 West Third, Suite 240E, Los Angeles, CA 90048, USA
* Corresponding author.
E-mail address: mckennar@cshs.org

Thorac Surg Clin 25 (2015) 349–354
http://dx.doi.org/10.1016/j.thorsurg.2015.04.004
1547-4127/15/$ – see front matter

mediastinum. In addition, if preoperative work-up proves that the IMA graft is occluded, lysis of adhesions can be performed without concern for compromising the graft.

The risk of injury to coronary bypass grafts in general thoracic operations is not well defined. The literature until recently consisted of only a few case reports describing open techniques of preserving a small amount of lung parenchyma adherent to the LIMA pedicle to minimize the risk of injury to the bypass graft.[6–9] A 2003 case report of an open operation by Halkos and colleagues[6] described the technique of sequentially stapling across the adherent pulmonary parenchyma to detach the left upper lobe from the mediastinum and LIMA graft. The operation was performed with a posterolateral thoracotomy. They reported no complications of infection or tumor recurrence in five patients when this technique was used. A similar approach was reported by Singhatanadgige and colleagues[9] in 2006. Santini and colleagues[8] in 2008 describe the same operation; however, instead of a stapling device, a Ligasure (Covidien, Mineapolis, MN, USA) bipolar tissue sealing system was used to divide the parenchyma and adhesions. All of these case reports involved open operations and until 2014, the technique had not been described in the literature via a VATS approach.

Recently, this technique was reported in a retrospective study of 14 patients who underwent VATS left upper lobectomy after coronary artery bypass grafting (CABG) using a LIMA graft.[10] These patients underwent VATS with full mobilization of the lung, except for the area adherent to the chest wall, mediastinum, and LIMA graft. Sequential stapling transected the lung parenchyma, while leaving some lung tissue attached to the LIMA graft to avoid any actual dissection of the graft and minimize possibly injuring the graft. There was no specific protocol for the preoperative evaluation of these patients, although in some cases the work-up included cardiac catheterization (N = 3), transthoracic echocardiography (N = 3), treadmill stress test (N = 2), and stress echocardiography (N = 2) with one occluded LIMA graft identified preoperatively. Compared with other patients who underwent VATS lobectomy over the same time period, but without a history of LIMA grafts, the patients who had LIMA grafts experienced no statistical difference in perioperative mortality, postoperative length of stay, rate of conversion to thoracotomy, complication rate or cardiac complication rate, and no patient in the LIMA graft group experienced evidence of perioperative cardiac ischemia. Significant differences were demonstrated in the LIMA graft group with respect to the need for blood transfusion (3.3% vs 14.3%; $P = .04$), empyema (0.7% vs 14.3%; $P<.01$), and takeback for bleeding (0.4% vs 7.1%; $P = .003$). The authors postulated that the increased incidence of empyema could be caused by the presumed devitalized lung parenchyma left attached to the LIMA graft, but no definitive conclusions could be demonstrated. At 60-months follow-up, no recurrences were found in the residual lung parenchyma around the LIMA graft.

To better characterize the hospital course for patients undergoing VATS lobectomy after sternotomy for cardiac surgery, the authors retrospectively reviewed their patient database of 2684 VATS lobectomies (from 1992 through 2012) to identify 87 patients who underwent VATS lobectomy after heart surgery.[11] Their cardiac surgical histories included CABG (64), valve replacement or repair (12), CABG and valve replacement (6), and transplant (5). There were 70 patients who underwent CABG and one who underwent CABG before a cardiac transplant. Eighteen patients had confirmed ipsilateral IMA grafts, although data regarding the details of the heart surgery were not complete, so additional patients likely had ipsilateral IMA grafts. There was one intraoperative injury to a LIMA graft. The operation was converted to a muscle-sparing thoracotomy by enlarging the utility incision, and the arterial graft was repaired primarily; after the repair, Doppler examination confirmed flow within the graft. The patient had no hemodynamic or ST changes intraoperatively and did not experience a myocardial infarction (MI). The technique of dividing the pulmonary parenchyma that is adherent to the mediastinum as described in this article was not used in the patient who suffered the LIMA injury.

Comparison of outcomes of all our VATS lobectomy patients with and without history of sternotomy for cardiac surgery did demonstrate significant differences between the groups. Patients with a history of cardiac surgery had an increased risk of airleak, acute respiratory distress syndrome, atrial fibrillation, blood transfusion, chest tube drainage greater than 6 days, empyema, mortality, overall complications, renal failure, and return to the operating room for bleeding. **Table 1** compares the incidence of perioperative events in the two groups of patients. There was no difference in the rate of MI or mortality caused by MI. These data demonstrate the difficulties in surgical and medical management of these complicated patients.

Although the technique discussed in this article evolved to safely manage adhesions between the lung and IMA grafts, it can also be used in any patient who has had a sternotomy. If adhesions to the mediastinum are too dense for safe dissection or if

Table 1
Outcomes of VATS lobectomy patients with and without history of sternotomy for cardiac surgery

Complication Rates	History of Cardiac Surgery via Sternotomy, % (N = 88)	No History of Sternotomy,% (N = 2684)	*P*
Air leak	14.77	5.10	.0007
Acute respiratory distress syndrome	2.27	0.07	.0057
Atrial fibrillation	9.09	3.70	.0243
Blood transfusion	13.64	2.40	<.0001
Chest tube drainage >6 d	18.18	5.80	<.0001
Empyema	3.40	0.50	.0152
Mortality	5.68	0.80	.0011
Mortality caused by MI	1.13	0.11	.1211
MI	2.27	0.48	.08
No complication	50.00	74.00	<.0001
Pneumonia	2.27	1.10	.2701
Readmission with 30 d of discharge	3.40	1.41	.1468
Renal failure	5.68	0.56	.0003
Return to operating room for bleeding	3.40	0.56	.0179

From Serna-Gallegos D, Merry H, Soukiasian HJ, et al. Video assisted thoracic surgery in patients with previous sternotomy and cardiac surgery. 2014. Unpublished data submitted for consideration for presentation at the AATS Annual meeting. Seattle, WA. April 25–29, 2015.

the lung is stuck to other vital structures, which would be unsafe to manipulate, the technique described here can be an important tool in the armamentarium of the general thoracic surgeon.

SURGICAL TECHNIQUE

Preoperative Planning

Preoperative planning may include the following:

- Obtain operative report of cardiac operation
- Review images of most recent cardiac catheterization
- Possible cardiac MRI or CT angiography of heart to better define the location of IMA graft and its patency
- Cardiac clearance

Preparation and Patient Positioning

Preparation and patient positioning include the following:

- Lateral decubitus positioning with slight posterior tilt.
- A beanbag used for positioning and the patient is taped down to the table at the level of the anterior superior iliac spine.
- Arms are at 90° with elbows bent in praying position with two pillows between the arms, and padding on elbow of arm on armboard minimizes risk of ulnar nerve injury.
- Anterior superior iliac crest should be positioned at the break of the table and table should be flexed to move hips out of the way so that the hips do not compromise camera mobility. This also helps to open up the rib interspaces.
- Monitors are placed at head of the bed for an unobscured view.
- Positioning usually does not need to be adjusted for intraoperative crisis.
- Conversion to thoracotomy can be performed through a posterolateral thoracotomy or extension of the utility incision to make a muscle-sparing thoracotomy.

Monitoring

Monitoring is by radial arterial line. Central venous catheter is not routinely used.

Surgical Approach

Poststernotomy adhesions are concentrated along the mediastinum and posteriorly by the diaphragm. If the adhesions are more diffuse or if a VATS approach cannot provide adequate visualization of the adhesions and the mediastinum, conversion to a thoracotomy may be necessary.

However, through the 2-cm incision in the sixth intercostal space in the mid-clavicular line, adhesions can be lysed toward the diaphragm to allow placement of a trocar and thoracoscope in the posterior axillary line to better visualize adhesions for lysis. That maneuver usually creates enough space to then lyse the remainder of the adhesions.

Surgical Procedure

Incision placement

- First incision is 2 cm in the sixth intercostal interspace (one interspace below inframammary fold) as anteriorly and inferiorly as possible. Dissection through chest wall tunnels posteriorly from the skin incision so instruments are directed toward the major fissure and away from the pericardium.
- Trocar and thoracoscope go through the eighth interspace in the posterior axillary line. This incision is tunneled slightly superiorly to decrease the torque placed on the intercostal nerve.
- Next, the location of the utility incision is determined by the pulmonary vein; for an upper or middle lobe, the incision is made directly up from the vein, starting at the anterior edge of the latissimus dorsi and is continued 4 to 6 cm anteriorly. A soft tissue protector or a Weitlaner retractor is placed in the utility incision to keep the soft tissues open so that suction can be used in the chest without re-expanding the lung.
- If conversion to thoracotomy is needed the utility incision can be extended to 10 cm for a muscle-sparing thoracotomy.
- For upper lobectomies, a 1-cm incision is placed in the auscultatory triangle. This incision can be used for lung retraction and staplers for division of upper lobe vessels.

Camera and visualization considerations

- A 5-mm thoracoscope is used because it provides adequate visualization and decreases the torque placed on the intercostal nerves by a 10-mm scope.
- A 30-degree scope allows the surgeon to look around structures better than a 0-degree scope.
- In general, a panoramic view with the thoracoscope provides the best view to assess the general anatomy. Especially when dissecting with electrocautery or dissecting near such structures as an IMA graft, the wide view (maximal zoom out) allows for a safer assessment of the anatomy and progress of the operation.

Safe dissection of adhesions by internal mammary artery

The initial step is to assess the extent of adhesions from the previous sternotomy. These adhesions can range from thin transparent film-like adhesions to dense adhesions that stick the lung parenchyma anteriorly in the mediastinum as seen in **Fig. 1**.

Division of adhesions to mediastinum

The division of the adhesions between the lung and mediastinum can be performed as an initial effort to separate the lung before hilar dissection. If adhesions are thin and film-like they can be safely divided using a harmonic scalpel as in **Fig. 2**.

If adhesions are dense and the dissection is not safe anteriorly near the IMA, first dissect along the mediastinum away from the IMA graft and closer to the hilum of the lung. The adhesions are usually not as dense by the phrenic nerve and the hilum so the lung can be separated from the mediastinum in that area. That dissection helps to create a tunnel between the lung and the mediastinum through which a stapler anvil can be passed to transect the pulmonary tissue adherent to the IMA graft (**Fig. 3**).

The stapler can then fire across the lung parenchyma close to the mediastinum, but away from the IMA. That maneuver finishes separating the lung from the mediastinum. This leaves a small amount of lung parenchyma attached to the IMA and separated from the rest of the upper lobe.

Preoperative imaging studies may provide some guidance as to the location of the IMA graft within the mediastinum. Intraoperatively, this relationship

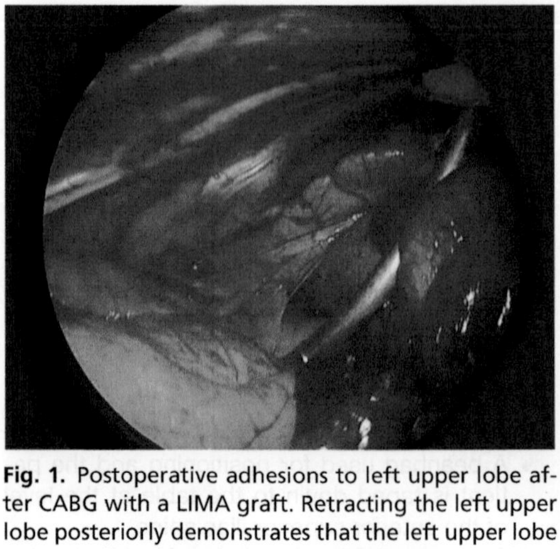

Fig. 1. Postoperative adhesions to left upper lobe after CABG with a LIMA graft. Retracting the left upper lobe posteriorly demonstrates that the left upper lobe is more adherent to the anterior mediastinum and less by the hilum.

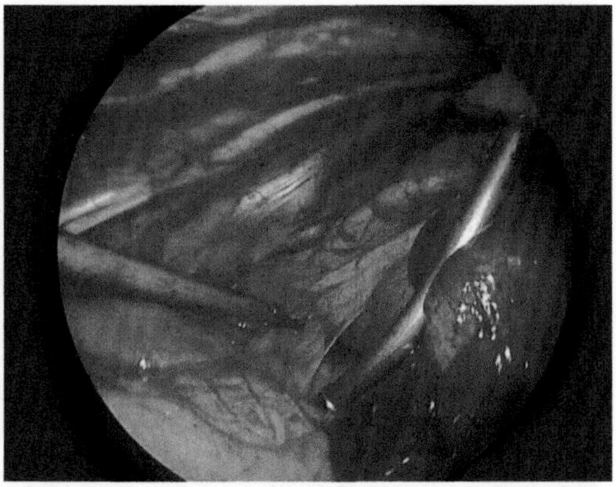

Fig. 2. The harmonic scalpel divides the filmy adhesions between lung parenchyma and pericardium. The left upper lobe is retracted superiorly and posteriorly toward the apex of the left hemithorax. One should be careful about the collateral thermal spread of the instrumentation.

to the mediastinum can be used as a guide to divide the adhesions safely. If there is confusion as to the location of the patent graft intraoperatively, Doppler can be used to identify the IMA graft. **Fig. 4** shows the adhesed lung parenchyma after a single firing of the 45-mm staple load.

Once the adhesions are completely divided there is a small amount of residual lung parenchyma that is left adherent to the mediastinum to preserve the IMA graft as in **Fig. 5**. Blood supply through the adhesions keeps that small amount of lung parenchyma viable. Our patients have not experienced an empyema from this technique.

Management of injury to internal mammary artery graft

Most importantly these complicated procedures should only be performed at institutions that have a cardiac surgery team that can perform cardiac bypass and revise the graft or redo CABG if needed. Conversion to thoracotomy can be performed to provide improved exposure of injury to the IMA graft, as needed.

When bleeding occurs, a sponge stick or Ratek gauze places pressure to control the bleeding, as a game plan is made to solve the problem. If the graft is visible and amenable to primary repair, it can be performed with polypropylene suture. Continual bleeding not amenable to primary repair could potentially necessitate the need for cardiac surgical intervention and possibly cardiac bypass, although we have not seen that.

Postoperative electrocardiograms and troponins are checked, if indicated. These tests are not routinely checked if the clinical course and physiology do not suggest any impairment. A cardiologist is consulted to help with postoperative cardiac management.

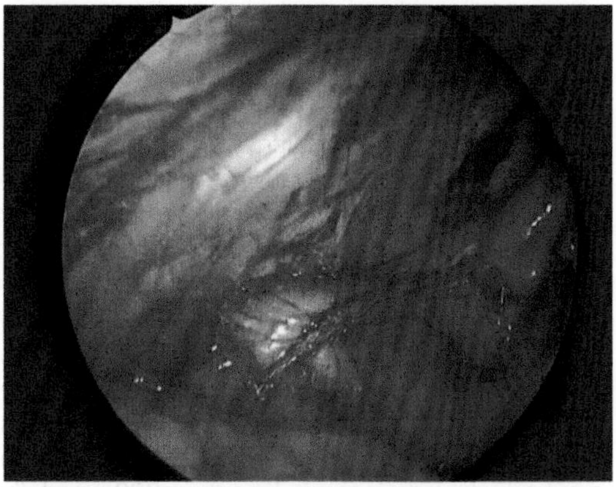

Fig. 4. After firing the stapler once across the lung, a small amount of residual parenchyma is left attached to the mediastinum to preserve the IMA graft.

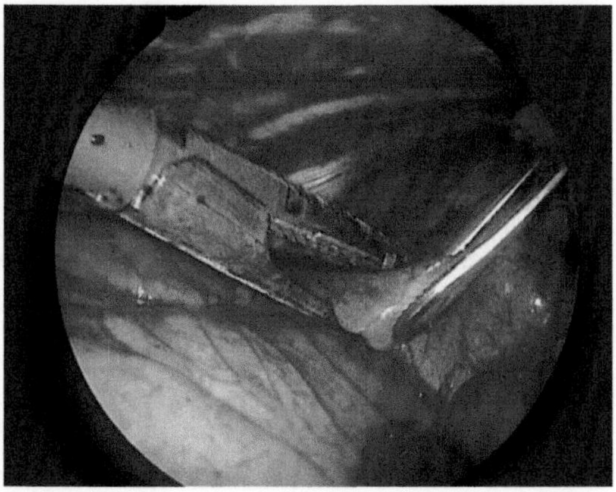

Fig. 3. Division of lung parenchyma that is adherent to the mediastinum and is in relatively close proximity to the LIMA graft.

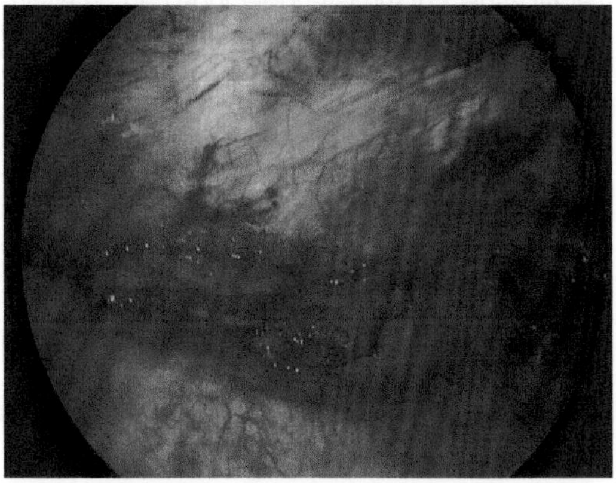

Fig. 5. Completion of division of the adhesions. The lung is now fully separated from the mediastinum and only a small amount of lung parenchyma remains attached to the mediastinum.

IMMEDIATE POSTOPERATIVE CARE

Postoperatively, patients are monitored with telemetry on the floor or intensive care unit, as indicated. Patients are not routinely sent to the intensive care unit. Preoperative medications are ordered and monitored by the cardiologist throughout the hospital stay, with antiplatelet or anticoagulation medications started on postoperative Day 1 if the patient is not bleeding. Patients are ambulated on postoperative Day 0 or 1 when they have awakened from anesthesia. Aggressive pulmonary toilet and incentive spirometry begins immediately postoperatively. Chest tubes are removed when drainage is less than 300 mL daily and there is no airleak.

REHABILITATION AND RECOVERY

If no cardiac complications have occurred, the patient should undergo routine rehabilitation and recovery with early ambulation and return to activities.

SUMMARY

VATS lobectomies can be safely performed in patients with ipsilateral IMA grafts in institutions where adequate resources exist for management of complications including cardiopulmonary bypass and redo CABG. Compared with patients without a history of median sternotomy for cardiac surgery, patients with that history have a higher risk of overall complications, airleak, acute respiratory distress syndrome, atrial fibrillation, blood transfusion, chest tube drainage greater than 6 days, empyema, mortality, renal failure, and return to the operating room for bleeding. When reviewing the chest CT, if contrast was used, the patency and location of the IMA graft and the medial aspect of the left upper lobe can be evaluated to determine if they are located in the anterior mediastinum. The technique of a stapler transecting lung parenchyma to leave a small amount of residual lung tissue with preservation of the IMA graft can be performed via VATS to separate the remainder of the upper lobe parenchyma. This technique allows a safe anatomic resection, while minimizing risks associated with manipulation of or dissecting near IMA grafts.

The incidence of injury to IMA grafts is low and can usually be managed with primary repair if the injury does not involve a complete transection of the vessel; cardiac surgical teams can be mobilized to aid in repair as needed.

REFERENCES

1. Whitson BA, Groth SS, Duval SJ, et al. Surgery for early-stage non-small cell lung cancer: a systematic review of the video-assisted thoracoscopic surgery versus thoracotomy approaches to lobectomy. Ann Thorac Surg 2008;86(6):2008–16 [discussion: 16–8].
2. Shaw JP, Dembitzer FR, Wisnivesky JP, et al. Video-assisted thoracoscopic lobectomy: state of the art and future directions. Ann Thorac Surg 2008;85(2): S705–9.
3. Boffa DJ, Allen MS, Grab JD, et al. Data from the Society of Thoracic Surgeons general thoracic surgery database: the surgical management of primary lung tumors. J Thorac Cardiovasc Surg 2008;135(2): 247–54.
4. Gillinov AM, Casselman FP, Lytle BW, et al. Injury to a patent left internal thoracic artery graft at coronary reoperation. Ann Thorac Surg 1999;67(2):382–6.
5. Imran Hamid U, Digney R, Soo L, et al. Incidence and outcome of re-entry injury in redo cardiac surgery: benefits of preoperative planning. Eur J Cardiothorac Surg 2015;47(5):819–23.
6. Halkos ME, Sherman AJ, Miller JI Jr. Preservation of the lima pedicle after cardiac surgery in left upper lobectomy. Ann Thorac Surg 2003;76(1):280–1.
7. Funaki S, Inoue M, Shigemura N, et al. Thoracoscopic lobectomy for lung cancer after coronary artery bypass grafting using internal thoracic artery. Interact Cardiovasc Thorac Surg 2012;15(5):928–9.
8. Santini M, Fiorello A, Vicidomini G, et al. The use of LigaSure for preservation of a previous coronary artery bypass graft by using the left internal thoracic artery in a left upper lobectomy. J Thorac Cardiovasc Surg 2008;136(1):222–3.
9. Singhatanadgige S, Sindhvanada W, Kittayarak C. Left upper lobectomy after CABG with the left internal mammary artery graft. J Med Assoc Thai 2006; 89(6):887–9.
10. Shah AA, Worni M, Onaitis MW, et al. Thoracoscopic left upper lobectomy in patients with internal mammary artery coronary bypass grafts. Ann Thorac Surg 2014;98(4):1207–12.
11. Serna-Gallegos D, Merry H, Soukiasian HJ, et al. Video assisted thoracic surgery in patients with previous sternotomy and cardiac surgery. 2014. Unpublished data submitted for consideration for presentation at the AATS Annual meeting. Seattle, WA. April 25–29, 2015.

Postlobectomy Early Complications

Elena Ziarnik, MD[a], Eric L. Grogan, MD, MPH[b,*]

KEYWORDS

• Air leak • Atrial fibrillation • Pneumonia/mucous plugging • Right middle lobe torsion • Hemorrhage • Chylothorax • Nerve injury

KEY POINTS

- Immediate postoperative complications (ie, those occurring within 48 hours of the operation) are common after lobectomy.
- Prevention strategies in the operating room and in the early postoperative setting can minimize these risks.
- A proactive approach may minimize the long-term sequelae of postoperative complications.

INTRODUCTION

The most effective management of postoperative crises is prevention, which starts with preoperative preparation and patient screening. There are many factors that can be controlled and improved by the patient, including, but not limited to, smoking cessation, cardiopulmonary rehabilitation, and teaching/setting perioperative expectations. Equally important is patient selection, which is influenced by pulmonary function tests, cardiopulmonary reserve, and preexisting comorbidities. After the operation, the care team can also greatly improve outcomes with aggressive cardiopulmonary therapies, ambulation, vigilant monitoring, and frequent assessments of the patient. Even when all of these guidelines are followed, not all early complications can be avoided.

A recent review of the National Cancer Database by Rosen and colleagues[1] found a 2.6% mortality from lobectomy. Morbidity associated with lobectomy is 10% to 50%, and increases in the elderly.[2] The population being treated by thoracic surgeons continues to age and the complexity of the operations is increasing as neoadjuvant therapies become more prevalent. Early postoperative crises after lobectomy occur, necessitating prompt and effective management strategies. The most common complications after pulmonary resection are listed in **Table 1**. This article focuses on the early complications after lobectomy.[3]

This article defines early postoperative crisis as one that develops within 48 hours of the operation.

AIR LEAK

Prolonged air leak is the most common complication after pulmonary resection, with a reported incidence of 15% to 18%.[4] Prolonged air leak is defined as a leak lasting more than 7 days after pulmonary resection. Cerfolio and colleagues[5,6] reported an incidence of 25% on postoperative day

Dr E.L. Grogan is a recipient of the Department of Veterans' Affairs, Veterans Health Administration, Health Services Research and Development Service Career Development Award (10–024). The views expressed in this article are those of the authors and do not necessarily represent the views of the Department of Veterans' Affairs.

[a] Department of Thoracic Surgery, Vanderbilt University Medical Center, 1313 21st Avenue South, Nashville, TN 37232, USA; [b] Department of Thoracic Surgery, Tennessee Valley Healthcare System, Nashville Campus, Vanderbilt University Medical Center, 609 Oxford House, 1313 21st Avenue South, Nashville, TN 37232, USA
* Corresponding author.
E-mail address: eric.grogan@vanderbilt.edu

Thorac Surg Clin 25 (2015) 355–364
http://dx.doi.org/10.1016/j.thorsurg.2015.04.003
1547-4127/15/$ – see front matter Published by Elsevier Inc.

Table 1
Postlobectomy morbidity and mortality in the ACOSOG Z0030 trial

Complication	% of Patients
Mortality	1.4
Reoperation for bleeding	1.5
Prolonged air leak	7.6
Empyema	1.1
Pneumonia	2.5
Bronchopleural fistula	0.5
Atelectasis	6.4
ARDS	0.7
Atrial fibrillation	14.4

Total number of patients 766.

Abbreviation: ARDS, acute respiratory distress syndrome.

Data from Allen MS, Darling GE, Pechet TT, et al. Morbidity and mortality of major pulmonary resections in patients with early-stage lung cancer: initial results of the randomized, prospective ACOSOG Z0030 trial. Ann Thorac Surg 2006;81(3):1013–9.

1 and 20% on postoperative day 2. There are many techniques available to reduce parenchymal air leaks postoperatively and a variety of factors that influence any given patient's propensity for developing an air leak. Patient factors that increase the risk of developing an air leak include emphysematous lungs, larger parenchymal resection and therefore less parenchymal apposition to chest wall, and inadequate drainage of air by thoracostomy tubes.

PREVENTION STRATEGIES

Bronchial Stump Buttressing with a Muscle Flap

In patients with an infected pleural space or who are on chronic immunosuppression, coverage of the stump with vascularized muscle may prevent bronchial stump breakdown.[7] The intercostal muscle is an excellent coverage option and is harvested from the intercostal space on entry into the chest at the level of the thoracotomy. It is important to plan ahead, because this muscle needs to be harvested before placing the rib spreader in an open operation to prevent crushing the vascular supply. Dissection is begun on the inferior rib and the muscle is mobilized using a periosteal elevator posteriorly to the paraspinous muscle. Attention is then turned to the superior rib, taking great care to maintain the neurovascular bundle. The muscle is divided as far anteriorly as possible before encountering or endangering the internal mammary artery.

Pleural Tent

A pleural tent is developed by releasing the pleura from the chest wall over the top half of the hemithorax and allowing it to drape over the remaining lung.[8] The space above the pleura fills with blood and fluid, negating it as potential space and creating tissue apposition between the lung surface and the parietal pleura. The pleural tent is developed by incising the parietal pleura with electrocautery at the level of the access incision if the lobectomy was done thoracoscopically, or the thoracotomy incision if the lobectomy was done in an open manner. It is released bluntly from the chest wall, taking care to keep it intact. It is continued circumferentially in the chest until there is enough laxity that the pleura is in contact with the remaining inflated lung. The use of a pleural tent can be especially helpful in patients with emphysema, who are at a high risk of air leak, and those who will be left with a large potential pleural space after resection.

Suture Closure of Identified Leaks

Assessing lung parenchyma for air leak is possible by filling the thoracic cavity with sterile water and having the anesthesia team inflate the remaining lung.[9] Once a site of leak is identified, simple figure-of-eight suture closure of the visceral pleura can decrease postoperative air leak.

Buttressed Staple Line

There are a variety of products that can be used to buttress the staple line.[10–12] They are designed to work with major stapling devices. The most commonly used are bovine pericardium, polytetrafluoroethylene or a collagen matrix (Peri-Strips Dry). They are applied to the stapler before firing and function as full-length pledgets along the entirety of the staple line (**Fig. 1**).[13]

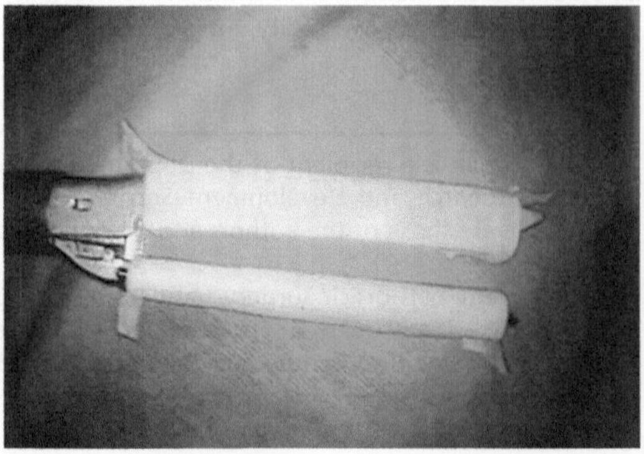

Fig. 1. Buttressed stapler.

Fissureless Operation

The pulmonary artery is frequently accessed via the fissure by dissecting free the parenchymal tissue with electrocautery or sharp dissection,[14] which can lead to air leaks from the divided parenchyma. In a fissureless lobectomy the pulmonary artery is exposed via the posterior hilum. As branches and the ongoing pulmonary artery are identified the parenchyma is stapled sequentially. This process allows all parenchyma to be stapled and divided, thus avoiding division with cautery or sharp dissection.[15]

Sealants

A Cochrane Database Review including 16 randomized trials with 1642 patients found that surgical sealants reduced postoperative air leaks and time to chest tube removal, but did not report a reduction in length of postoperative hospital stay.[16–18] A variety of sealants are available, including fibrin glue, cyanoacrylate, gelatin-resorcinol cross-linked with formaldehyde or glutaraldehyde, collagen, gelatin-based tissue adhesives, and polyurethane-based adhesives. They are activated by a variety of techniques and then applied to the divided parenchymal surface with an applicator in a stream or spray.

Expedited Liberation from Mechanical Ventilation

Most patients are extubated in the operating room after a lobectomy. Reducing the time on positive pressure ventilation and minimizing peak airway pressure decreases the incidence of postoperative alveolar air leak.

TREATMENT STRATEGIES

The timing and severity of the air leak affect treatment strategies.

Nonoperative Management

If the air leak is small and expiratory, chest tube management is the first step in management. Cerfolio and colleagues[6] published a randomized study in which chest tubes were continued on suction or placed to water seal on postoperative day 2. By postoperative day 3 the leak had resolved in 67% of patients on water seal, and only 7% on suction. It is advised that air leaks are best treated with water seal of the chest tube as long as a pneumothorax does not develop or increase and respiratory function is not compromised. Air leaks that do not resolve should be placed to one-way valve for discharge with the goal of tube removal in clinic at follow-up.

Operative Management

If the air leak develops suddenly or increases to a continuous leak, a high index of suspicion is necessary for a bronchopleural fistula (BPF). The risk is highest after a pneumonectomy (right greater than left [8.6% vs 2.3% respectively]).[19] BPF development after lobectomy in the first 48 hours is rare. Factors that increase the risk of BPF development include immunocompromise, neoadjuvant radiation, infection (uncommon as an early postoperative issue), steroid use, diabetes,[20] skeletonizing the bronchial stump with dissection, and leaving a long bronchial stump.[21] Prevention of BPF is paramount because of high mortalities if it occurs.[19] Particularly with pneumonectomy, the bronchial stump should be covered with autologous tissue. Tissue options include pericardium, mediastinal fat pad, intercostal muscle flap, parietal pleura, and azygous vein.[21]

Development of a BPF as an early postoperative complication after lobectomy is a surgical problem that is solved by a return to the operating room. Diagnosis of a BPF can be clinical, but is confirmed bronchoscopically. If the bronchoscopy is negative and the index of suspicion remains high, a ventilation perfusion scan can be performed, which shows the tagged gas exiting the pleural space through the chest tube.

In the operating room the chest is reentered through the incisions made during the primary operation. Depending on the initial approach an intercostal muscle flap can be harvested as described earlier on reexploration. If the intercostal muscle is not viable from prior retraction or injury, attention can be turned to a vascularized mediastinal fat pad or the latissimus or serratus muscles. The pleural space is cleared of fluid and debris and the bronchial stump is identified and debrided. If the stump is healthy, primary repair can be attempted; of greater importance is well-vascularized autologous tissue coverage. The covered stump needs to be tested for any remaining leak before chest closure.

Pneumonia/Mucous Plugging

Pneumonia is a significant concern for thoracic surgeons, with a reported incidence of up to 6% in some studies.[22] Patients are at increased risk after chest surgery for poor pulmonary hygiene, which can lead to the development of atelectasis and progression to pneumonia and/or mucous plugging. Atelectasis causes a ventilation/perfusion mismatch that results in hypoxemia and respiratory decline. Factors that increase the risk of atelectasis include poor cough, poor pain control, impaired pulmonary function at baseline, and anatomic factors such as chest wall or diaphragm dysfunction.

PREVENTION STRATEGIES

Chest Physiotherapy

Chest physiotherapy (CPT), including coughing and percussion, early ambulation, and incentive spirometry, is the standard approach for postoperative prophylaxis against atelectasis and sputum retention.

Aggressive Strategies

Nasotracheal suctioning, intermittent positive pressure ventilation, inhaled mucolytics, and bedside percussion may become necessary in patients with recalcitrant mucous plugging and atelectasis to encourage and produce an effective cough.

Pain Control

Poor postoperative pain control decreases patients' ability to participate in the standard CPT activities, which impairs their ability to clear their secretions. The use of narcotic pain medication can improve pain control, but may lead to altered mental status and impaired ability to clear secretions, and so the cycle continues. Debate exists over the optimal pain control strategy. There is good evidence that video-assisted thoracoscopic surgery causes less postoperative pain than open thoracotomies.[23] Epidural analgesia, intercostal nerve blocks, and patient-controlled intravascular analgesia (PCA) are the most common methods used. Each method has advantages and disadvantages. Epidural analgesia provides excellent pain relief, but carries the risk of bradycardia, hypotension, and urinary retention. Intercostal nerve blocks are short acting and may not be effective for the duration of patient recovery. PCAs are effective, but narcotics can lead to altered mental status and respiratory depression as described earlier.[24] Effective pain control is the goal and surgeon preference the deciding factor.

Smoking Cessation

Preoperative smoking cessation is a necessity to reduce sputum production and retention.[25] The risk of pulmonary complications are decreased the longer the interval between smoking cessation and surgery. The optimal timing of smoking cessation is not defined. Nakagawa and colleagues[26] found that a minimum of 4 weeks of smoking abstinence was needed to see a reduction in pulmonary complications. Other studies of cardiac patients concluded that 8 weeks of abstinence was best, but the cohort of patients is not entirely transferable.[27] Thoracic surgeons need to weigh the risk of smoking activity with delaying a cancer operation.

TREATMENT STRATEGIES

Antibiotic Treatment

Patients need to be treated for nosocomial bacteria with broad-spectrum antibiotics. The choice of antibiotic depends on the center. Before initiation of antibiotic therapy, blood and sputum cultures should be sent. The most effective way to obtain an airway specimen is by bronchoalveolar lavage from the airway with abnormality on chest radiograph or the airway with copious secretions on bronchoscopy.

Aggressive Chest Physiotherapy

Continuing standard postoperative CPT as noted earlier remains paramount. The addition of an expectorant and/or chest percussion can improve atelectasis. Therapeutic bronchoscopy to physically remove the mucous plug may also prove necessary. **Figs. 2–4** show the progression of atelectasis to mucous plugging and improvement after therapeutic bronchoscopy. The left lung does not return to its immediate postoperative expansion, but there is significant improvement after bronchoscopy.

Ventilatory Support

If the infection or effect on breathing mechanics is severe enough the patient may require respiratory support with the ventilator as the lung recovers. The goal of ventilator support is to allow effective gas exchange. There are multiple modes of

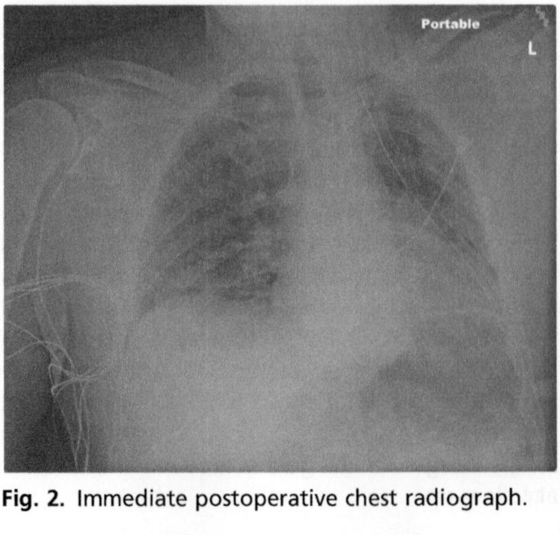

Fig. 2. Immediate postoperative chest radiograph.

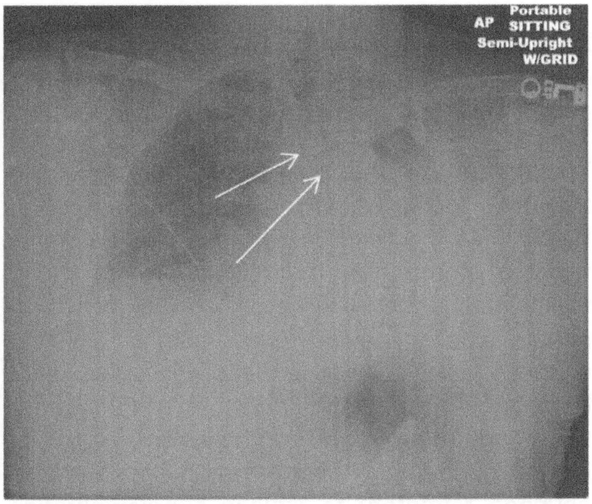

Fig. 3. Postoperative mucous plugging chest radiograph. Arrows denote mediastinal shift to the side of the collapse.

ventilation, the details of which are too broad for this article.

ATRIAL FIBRILLATION

Atrial fibrillation is the most common arrhythmia following pulmonary resection, with an incidence of 10% to 40% for all pulmonary resections, and 33% for lobectomy.[28] It most commonly occurs on postoperative day 2 or 3, but can occur at any time during recovery.[29] The mechanism of atrial fibrillation after noncardiac thoracic surgery is unknown, but there are multiple factors associated with developing postoperative atrial fibrillation. Risk factors include age greater than 70 years, amount of lung resected (right pneumonectomy carries the greatest risk), incision (clamshell), previous episode of congestive heart failure, male gender, prior arrhythmia, and blood transfusions.[30]

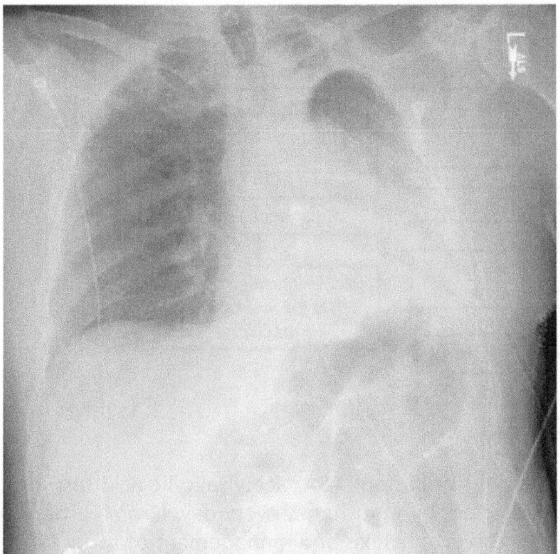

Fig. 4. Postbronchoscopy chest radiograph.

PREVENTION STRATEGIES

There are strategies to treat atrial fibrillation once it has occurred, but, much like air leaks, the best treatment is prevention. Management of fluid balance and electrolyte levels can decrease the incidence of atrial fibrillation. Multiple medications, including β-blockers, calcium-channel blockers, amiodarone, and digoxin have been used as prophylaxis against the development of atrial fibrillation.[31] Riber and colleagues[32] completed a meta-analysis and found amiodarone and magnesium sulfate to be the most effective and safest drugs as prophylaxis against postoperative atrial fibrillation. Amiodarone had a relative risk of 0.32 and a number needed to treat of 4.8. Overall, Riber and colleagues[32] found that the risk of postoperative atrial fibrillation reduced from 25.1% to 13.4% with the use of drug prophylaxis.

The Society of Thoracic Surgeons (STS) published a practice guideline in 2011 that included recommendations for atrial fibrillation prophylaxis.[33] Patients taking β-blockers preoperatively should continue postoperative administration, and should be titrated as blood pressure tolerates. In patients not taking β-blockers preoperatively, diltiazem and amiodarone should be considered for prophylaxis after a lobectomy. Flecainide and digoxin are not recommended as prophylaxis against postoperative atrial fibrillation.[33]

TREATMENT STRATEGIES

In patients who develop atrial fibrillation postoperatively, treatment is guided by their hemodynamic stability. Unstable patients need to be transferred to the intensive care unit and electrically cardioverted. The STS practice guidelines further state that hemodynamically stable patients should be chemically cardioverted with rate controlling medication for at least 24 hours. If chemical cardioversion is unsuccessful, electrical cardioversion can be used after 24 hours. The recommended agent of choice for rate control is a β1-selective blocker in the absence of moderate-severe chronic obstructive pulmonary disease (COPD) and diltiazem if moderate-severe COPD is present. For rhythm control, intravenous amiodarone or oral flecainide is recommended. Amiodarone should be avoided in ventilated patients, those who have had a pneumonectomy, or in patients with significant underlying lung disease because of pulmonary toxicity. Flecainide should be avoided with any underlying structural heart condition.[33] Nearly 50% of patients convert to normal sinus rhythm within 12 hours of rate control[34] with beta-blockade or calcium-channel blockers (**Fig. 5** provides an algorithm). If atrial fibrillation is recalcitrant to cardioversion or recurs for more than 48 hours, anticoagulation should be considered. In patients with 2 or more risk factors for a stroke (age >75 years, hypertension, impaired left ventricular function, prior stroke or transient ischemic attack), anticoagulation with warfarin is reasonable. For patients with fewer than 2 risk factors for stroke and patients considered not suitable for warfarin, aspirin (325 mg daily) is reasonable.

RIGHT MIDDLE LOBE TORSION

Postoperative lobar torsion is a rare but life-threatening complication after pulmonary resection, with a prevalence of 0.09% to 0.4%.[35] Torsion of the right middle lobe (RML) accounts for 70% of cases in the literature. Twisting of the lobe on its pedicle can lead to ischemia, pulmonary infarction, and gangrene unless treated promptly. Factors that increase the risk of torsion include a complete fissure, lack of adhesions, and complete mobilization of remaining lung.[36]

PREVENTION STRATEGIES

Torsion can be prevented with simple tacking of the RML to the remaining right lower or upper lobes.[37] Tacking can be performed with a simple figure-of-eight suture through the visceral pleura to maintain lobar orientation or with an endoscopic stapling device (pneumopexy).[38] Neither of these techniques is required and visualization of lobar expansion at the conclusion of the operation is adequate. Signs and symptoms of torsion include sudden and unexplained dyspnea and tachypnea refractory to oxygen supplementation, early high fever, and copious secretions (hemorrhagic or clear).[39] Chest radiograph may show sudden opacification of previously expanded lobe (**Figs. 6** and **7**).

Diagnosis is confirmed with bronchoscopy, with visualization of a compressed lobar bronchus with a classic fish-mouth appearance.[40] Computed tomography (CT) scan with contrast shows loss of blood flow and bronchial cutoff. Transesophageal echo may show right heart strain and turbulent

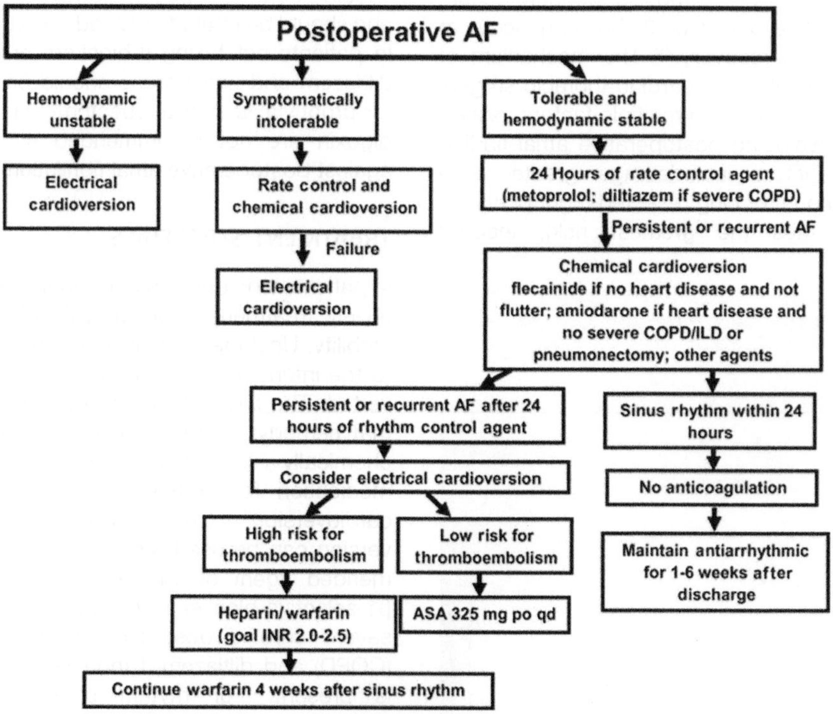

Fig. 5. Management of postoperative atrial fibrillation. AF, atrial fibrillation; ASA, acetylsalicylic acid (aspirin); ILD, interstitial lung disease; INR, International Normalized Ratio; po, by mouth; qd, every day. (*From* Fernando HC, Jaklitsch MT, Walsh GL, et al. The STS practice guideline on the prophylaxis and management of atrial fibrillation associated with general thoracic surgery: an executive summary. Ann Thorac Surg 2011;92:1150; with permission.)

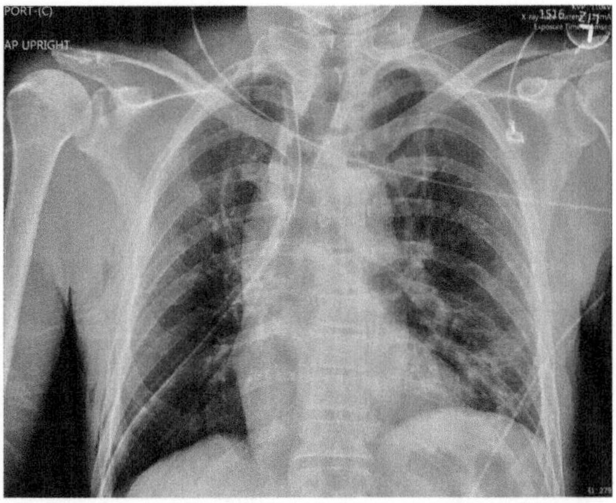

Fig. 6. Immediate postoperative chest radiograph.

flow, and possibly thrombus, in the pulmonary vein. A high index of suspicion is important and can improve patient outcomes if reoperation is undertaken before ischemia or gangrene occur.

TREATMENT STRATEGIES

Treatment of lobar torsion necessitates a completion lobectomy if ischemic necrosis or gangrene is present. It is important to evaluate for venous thrombosis before untwisting the lobe to avoid a potentially fatal stroke.[41] This evaluation can be accomplished with CT angiography preoperatively and/or intraoperative transesophageal echo. Reexpansion pulmonary edema can also occur and may require prolonged mechanical ventilation and frequent therapeutic bronchoscopy.[42] If the torsion is incomplete it may be possible to preserve the twisted lobe. Pexy of the lobe to the adjacent lobe should be performed with a stapler or suture.

HEMORRHAGE

The incidence of postoperative bleeding after lobectomy requiring at least 4 units of packed red

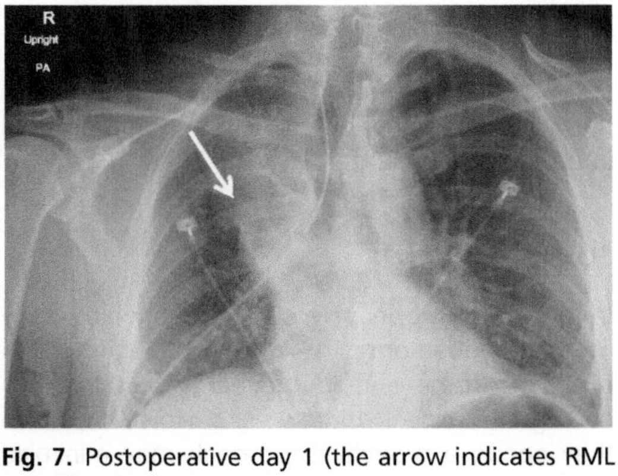

Fig. 7. Postoperative day 1 (the arrow indicates RML opacification).

blood cells was found to be 2.9%.[43] If the patient drains greater than 1 L in 1 hour or 200 mL/h for 4 hours, coagulation tests need to be checked, and, if normal, reexploration is indicated. Meticulous inspection of all dissection fields and incision sites before closing and ensuring hemostasis can help avoid postoperative hemorrhage that requires reexploration. There are multiple sources for postoperative bleeding. Sirbu and colleagues[44] reported the possible sources as mediastinal or bronchial vessel (23%), intercostal vessel (17%), pulmonary vessel (17%), and unidentifiable (41%). A systematic approach is best to inspect all areas of the thorax when reexploration is undertaken for hemothorax, including the lymph node beds, the inferior pulmonary ligament, and all staple lines. A dental mirror can be useful to get a full view of all aspects of incisions and chest tube sites.

CHYLOTHORAX

Chylothorax occurs because of injury of the thoracic duct. The incidence of chylothorax with pulmonary resection is 0.7% to 2%.[45] Aggressive mediastinal lymph node dissection and incomplete ligation of lymph node channels can lead to development of chylothorax. A diagnosis and treatment algorithm is shown in **Fig. 8**. Triglyceride level greater than 110 mg/dL and lymphocyte count greater than 90% are diagnostic. Attempts at conservative management for 5 to 7 days are accepted as long as the chest tube drainage decreases and the patient's nutritional balance can be maintained. Indications for surgical intervention include drainage of greater than 1500 mL/d in adults or greater than 100 mL/d in children for greater than 5 days, continued drainage for greater than 14 days total despite maximal medical management, or in patients after esophagectomy in whom drainage is more than 2 L/d for longer than 2 days.[46] Surgical management involves accessing the right chest and ligating the thoracic duct as low as possible. Direct repair is challenging because of difficulty in locating the injury directly.

NERVE INJURY

Phrenic Nerve

A variety of thoracic surgical procedures can lead to phrenic nerve injury. When focusing on lobectomy there is a higher risk of injury in the setting of adhesions to the pericardium and at the time of mediastinal lymph node dissection. Symptoms include dyspnea on exertion and diminished activity tolerance. Chest radiographs show an elevated

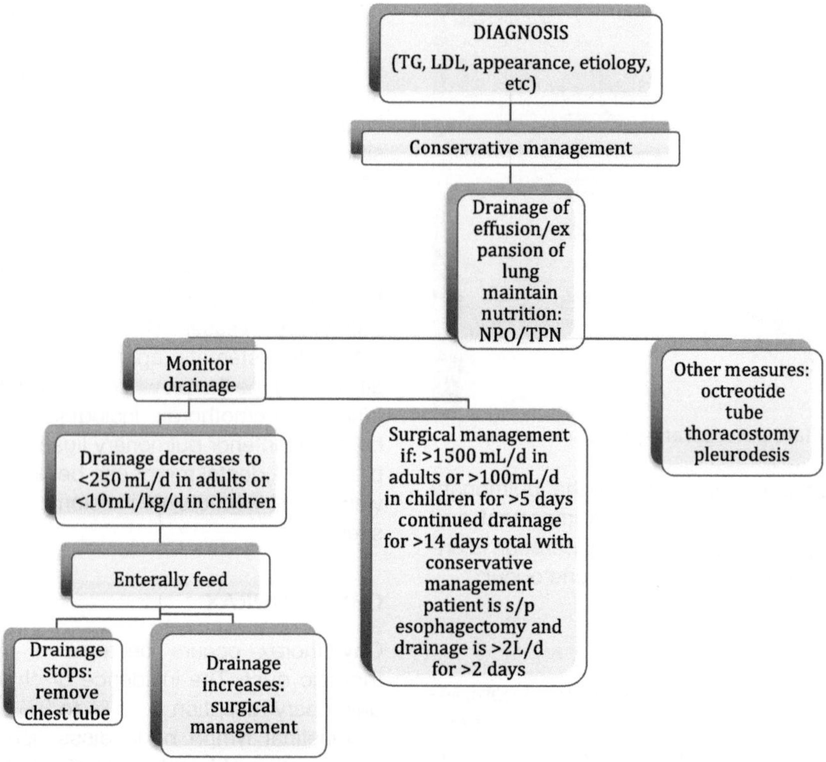

Fig. 8. Management algorithm for chylothorax. LDL, low-density lipoprotein; NPO, nothing per os; TG, triglyceride; TPN, total parenteral nutrition; s/p, status post. (*From* Ziarnik E, Nesbitt J. Chylothorax after esophageal surgery. In: Pawlik TM, Merchant N, Maithel SK, editors. Gastrointestinal, hepatobiliary, and pancreatic surgery: a procedure based guide for complex peri-operative situations and complications. New York: Springer Science and Business Media, in press.)

hemidiaphragm ipsilateral to the lobectomy. Diagnosis can be confirmed with a fluoroscopic sniff test, which shows paradoxic movement of the diaphragm on the side of injury. Depending on the degree of respiratory impairment, expectant management may be tolerated. If the patient is unable to maintain quality of life because of breathlessness, then diaphragm plication is indicated after 1 year with no return of function.

Recurrent Laryngeal Nerve

Injury to the recurrent laryngeal nerve can be detected early postoperatively and should be suspected in patients with weak voices, hoarseness, and weak cough. As patients are transitioned to a normal oral diet during recovery they may also experience aspiration after taking liquids. The symptoms are related to glottic incompetence and culminate in diminished airway protection and increased risk of pulmonary complications.[47] Diagnosis is made with direct fiberoptic laryngoscopy, which shows lack of movement of the effected cord with phonation. Once vocal cord dysfunction is confirmed the next step is to determine whether it is temporary or permanent. If the nerve was knowingly or purposefully injured during the conduct of the lobectomy, there is no need for further investigation. Treatment options include vocal cord injection or laryngeal framework surgery to medialize the paralyzed cord.[48] Early intervention most often involves collagen injection to medialize the cord and reestablish a competent glottis. Timing of intervention should be a joint decision between the thoracic surgeon and otolaryngologist. Early medialization can reduce pulmonary complications by reducing aspiration and improving cough and pulmonary toilet.[49]

SUMMARY

Immediate postoperative complications are common after lobectomy. Prevention strategies in the operating room and in the early postoperative setting can minimize these risks. However, when they occur, a proactive approach may minimize the long-term sequelae.

REFERENCES

1. Rosen JE, Hancock JG, Kim AW, et al. Predictors of mortality after surgical management of lung cancer in the National Cancer Database. Ann Thorac Surg 2014;98(6):1953–60.
2. Berry MF, Hanna J, Tong BC, et al. Risk factors for morbidity after lobectomy for lung cancer in elderly patients. Ann Thorac Surg 2009;88(4):1093–9.
3. Allen MS, Darling GE, Pechet TT, et al. Morbidity and mortality of major pulmonary resections in patients with early-stage lung cancer: initial results of the randomized, prospective ACOSOG Z0030 trial. Ann Thorac Surg 2006;81(3):1013–9.
4. Rice TW, Kirby TJ. Prolonged air leak. Chest Surg Clin North Am 1992;2:802–11.
5. Cerfolio RJ, Tummula RP, Holman WL, et al. A prospective algorithm for the management of air leaks after pulmonary resection. Ann Thorac Surg 1998;66:1726–31.
6. Cerfolio RJ, Bass CS, Katholi C. Prospective randomized trial compares suction versus water seal for air leaks. Ann Thorac Surg 2001;71:1613–7.
7. Babu AN, Mitchell JD. Technique of muscle flap harvest for intrathoracic use. Operative Tech in Thorac and Cardiovasc Surg 2010;15:41–52.
8. Uzzaman MM, Daniel RJ, Mhandu PC, et al. A meta-analysis assessing the benefits of concomitant pleural tent procedure after upper lobectomy. Ann Thorac Surg 2014;97:365–72.
9. Fell SC, DeCamp MM. Technical aspects of lobectomy. General Thoracic Surgery 2009;28:425–7.
10. Hazelrigg S, Boley TM, Naunheim KS, et al. Effect of bovine pericardial strips on air leak after stapled pulmonary resection. Ann Thorac Surg 1997;63:1573–5.
11. Stammberger UZ, Klepetko W, Stamatis G, et al. Buttressing the staple line in lung volume reduction surgery; a randomized three-center study. Ann Thorac Surg 2000;70:1820–5.
12. Itoh E, Matsuda S, Yaauchi K, et al. Synthetic absorbable film for prevention of air leaks after stapled pulmonary resection. J Biomed Mater Res 2000;53(6):640–5.
13. Fischel RJ, McKenna RJ. Bovine pericardium versus bovine collagen to buttress staples for lung reduction operations. Ann Thorac Surg 1998;65:217–9.
14. Gomez-Caro A, Roca-Calvo MJ, Lanzas JT, et al. The approach of the fused fissure with fissureless technique decreases the incidence of persistent air leak after lobectomy. Eur J Cardiothorac Surg 2007;31:203–8.
15. Temes RT, Willms CD, Santiago AE, et al. Fissureless lobectomy. Ann Thorac Surg 1998;65:282–4.
16. Malapert G, Hanna HA, Pages PB, et al. Surgical sealant for the prevention of prolonged air leak after lung resection; meta-analysis. Ann Thorac Surg 2010;90:1779–85.
17. Tansley P, Al-Mulhim F, Lim E, et al. A prospective, randomized, controlled trial of the effectiveness of Bioglue in treating alveolar air leaks. J Thorac Cardiovasc Surg 2006;132:105–12.
18. Belda-Sanchis J, Serra-Mitjan M, Iglesias Sentis M, et al. Surgical sealant for preventing air leaks after pulmonary resections in patients with lung cancer. Cochrane Database Syst Rev 2010;(1):CD003051.
19. Asamura H, Naruke T, Tsuchiya R, et al. Bronchopleural fistulas associated with lung cancer operations. Univariate and multivariate analysis of risk factors, management, and outcome. J Thorac Cardiovasc Surg 1992;104:1456–64.
20. Deschamps C, Bernard A, Nichols FC, et al. Empyema and bronchopleural fistula after pneumonectomy: factors affecting incidence. Ann Thorac Surg 2001;72:243–8.
21. Algar FJ, Alvarez A, Aranda JL, et al. Prediction of early bronchopleural fistula after pneumonectomy: a multivariate analysis. Ann Thorac Surg 2001;72:1662–7.
22. Deslauriers J, Ginsberg RJ, Piantadosi S, et al. Prospective assessment of 30-day operative morbidity for surgical resections in lung cancer. Chest 1994;106:329S–30S.
23. Nomori H, Horio H, Naruke T, et al. What is the advantage of a thoracoscopic lobectomy over a limited thoracotomy procedure for lung cancer surgery? Ann Thorac Surg 2001;72:879–84.
24. Luketich JD, Land SR, Sullivan EA. Thoracic epidural versus intercostal catheter plus patient-controlled analgesia: a randomized study. Ann Thorac Surg 2005;79:1845–50.
25. Bonde P, McManus K, McAnespie M, et al. Lung surgery: identifying the subgroup at risk for sputum retention. Eur J Cardiothorac Surg 2002;22:18–22.
26. Nakagawa M, Tanaka H, Tsukuma H, et al. Relationship between the duration of the preoperative smoke-free period and the incidence of postoperative pulmonary complications after pulmonary surgery. Chest 2001;120:705–10.
27. Warner MA, Divertie MB, Tinker JH. Preoperative cessation of smoking and pulmonary complications in coronary artery bypass patients. Anesthesiology 1984;60:380–3.
28. Roselli EE, Murthy SC, Rice TW, et al. Atrial fibrillation complicating lung cancer resection. J Thorac Cardiovasc Surg 2005;130:438–44.
29. Curtis JJ, Parker BM, McKenney CA, et al. Incidence and predictors of supraventricular dysrhythmias after pulmonary resection. Ann Thorac Surg 1998;66:1766–71.
30. Asamura H, Naruke T, Tsuchiya R, et al. What are the risk factors for arrhythmias after thoracic operations? A retrospective multivariate analysis of 267 consecutive thoracic operations. J Thorac Cardiovasc Surg 1993;106:1104–10.

31. Sedrakyan A, Treasure T, Browne J, et al. Pharmacologic prophylaxis for postoperative atrial tachyarrhythmia in general thoracic surgery: evidence from randomized clinical trials. J Thorac Cardiovasc Surg 2005;129:997–1005.
32. Riber LP, Larsen TB, Christensen TD, et al. Postoperative atrial fibrillation prophylaxis after lung surgery: systematic review and meta-analysis. Ann Thorac Surg 2014;98(6):1989–97.
33. Fernando HC, Jaklitsch MT, Walsh GL, et al. The STS practice guideline on the prophylaxis and management of atrial fibrillation associated with general thoracic surgery: an executive summary. Ann Thorac Surg 2011;92:1144–52.
34. Amar D. Postoperative atrial fibrillation. Heart Dis 2002;4:117–23.
35. Apostolakis E, Koletsis EN, Panagopoulos N, et al. Fatal stroke after completion pneumonectomy for torsion of left upper lobe following left lower lobectomy. J Cardiothorac Surg 2006;1:25.
36. Jones JM, Paxton LD, Graham AN. Acute postoperative lobar torsion associated with pulmonary arterial rupture. J Thorac Cardiovasc Surg 2003; 126(1):303.
37. Kutlu CA, Olgac G. Pleural flap to prevent lobar torsion: a novel technique. Eur J Cardiothorac Surg 2006;30:943–4.
38. Fell SC, DeCamp MM Jr. Chapter 28: technical aspects of lobectomy. General Thoracic Surgery 2005;7:425–7.
39. Ponn R. Complications of pulmonary resection. General Thoracic Surgery 2005;9:566–7.
40. Schamaun M. Postoperative pulmonary torsion: report of a case and survey of the literature including spontaneous and posttraumatic torsion. Thorac Cardiovasc Surg 1994;42:116–21.
41. Burri E, Duwe J, Kull C, et al. Pulmonary vein thrombosis after lower lobectomy of the left lung. J Cardiovasc Surg 2006;47:609–12.
42. Sakai M, Kurimori K, Seaki Y, et al. Video-assisted thoracoscopic conservative repair of postoperative lobar torsion. Ann Thorac Surg 2014;98:e119–21.
43. Harpole DH Jr, DeCamp MM Jr, Daley J, et al. Prognostics models of thirty-day mortality and morbidity after major pulmonary resection. J Thorac Cardiovasc Surg 1999;117:969–79.
44. Sirbu H, Busch T, Aleksic I, et al. Chest reexploration for complications after lung surgery. Thorac Cardiovasc Surg 1999;47:73–6.
45. Kutlu CA, Sayar A, Olgac G, et al. Chylothorax: a complication following lung resection in patients with NSCLC: chylothorax following lung resection. Thorac Cardiovasc Surg 2003;51:342–5.
46. Ziarnik E, Nesbitt J. Chylothorax after esophageal surgery. Gastrointestinal, hepatobiliary, and pancreatic surgery: a procedure based guide for complex peri-operative situations and complications, in press.
47. Murty GE, Kelly PJ, Bradley PJ. Tussometry: an objective assessment of vocal cord function. Ann Otol Rhinol Laryngol 1993;102:743–7.
48. Bhattacharyya N, Batirel H, Swanson SJ. Improved outcomes with early vocal fold medialization for vocal fold paralysis after thoracic surgery. Auris Nasus Larynx 2003;30:71–5.
49. Mom T, Filaire M, Advenioer D. Concomitant type 1 thyroplasty and thoracic operations for lung cancer: preventing respiratory complications associated with vagus or recurrent laryngeal nerve injury. J Thorac Cardiovasc Surg 2001;121:642–8.

Index

Note: Page numbers of article titles are in **boldface** type.

Thorac Surg Clin 25 (2015) 365–370
http://dx.doi.org/10.1016/S1547-4127(15)00041-9
1547-4127/15/$ – see front matter

R

S

Printed and bound by CPI Group (UK) Ltd, Croydon, CR0 4YY
03/10/2024
01040374-0007